Bringing Evidence Into Everyday Practice

Practical Strategies for Health Care Professionals

Second Edition

Bringing Evidence Into Everyday Practice

Practical Strategies for Health Care Professionals

Second Edition

WINNIE DUNN, PHD, OTR, FAOTA
DISTINGUISHED PROFESSOR
DEPARTMENT OF OCCUPATIONAL THERAPY
COLLEGE OF HEALTH SCIENCES
UNIVERSITY OF MISSOURI
COLUMBIA, MISSOURI

RACHEL PROFFITT, OTD, OTR/L
ASSOCIATE PROFESSOR
DEPARTMENT OF OCCUPATIONAL THERAPY
COLLEGE OF HEALTH SCIENCES
UNIVERSITY OF MISSOURI
COLUMBIA, MISSOURI

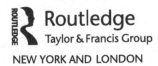

Routledge
Taylor & Francis Group

NEW YORK AND LONDON

Instructors: *Bringing Evidence Into Everyday Practice: Practical Strategies for Health Care Professionals, Second Edition,* includes ancillary materials specifically available for faculty use. Included is an *Instructor's Manual.* Please visit www.routledge.com/9781638220695 to obtain access.

First published 2024 by SLACK Incorporated

Published 2024 by Routledge
605 Third Avenue, New York, NY 10158

and by Routledge
4 Park Square, Milton Park, Abingdon, Oxon, OX14 4RN

Routledge is an imprint of the Taylor & Francis Group, an informa business

Library of Congress Control Number: 2023948176

Cover Artist: Tinhouse Design

ISBN: 9781638220695 (pbk)
ISBN: 9781003522782 (ebk)

DOI: 10.4324/9781003522782

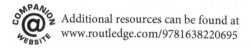 Additional resources can be found at
www.routledge.com/9781638220695

DEDICATION

We dedicate this book to the teachers and scholars who have paved the way in making occupational therapy an evidence-based profession. We are grateful for their forward thinking and perseverance in shaping our past, present, and future.

CONTENTS

Dedication. v
Master List of Worksheets viii
Acknowledgments xi
About the Authors xiii
Preface. xv
Introduction. xvii
How to Use This Book xxiii

Section I   Learning the Basics **1**
Unit 1   Introduction to Evidence-Based Practice. 3
Unit 2   Characterizing Responses to Evidence 9
Unit 3   Understanding and Using the Basic Parts of Research Articles 13

Section II   Practice Using Evidence to Design Best Practices **27**
Unit 4   Examining Evidence Related to Assistive Devices and
            Environmental Adaptations 29
Unit 5   Examining Evidence Related to the Use of Compensatory Strategies 37
Unit 6   Examining Evidence Related to Caregiving 43
Unit 7   Examining Evidence Related to Sensory Processing Patterns 49
Unit 8   Examining Evidence Related to Constraint-Induced
            Therapy Interventions 57
Unit 9   Examining Evidence Related to Upper Extremity Fractures. 65

**Section III   Expanding Your Knowledge and Skills
                 for Evidence-Based Practice** **75**
Unit 10   Understanding Summary and Meta-Analysis Articles 77
Unit 11   Examining Evidence Related to Emerging and Controversial Practices 89
Unit 12   Creating Evidence Within Your Own Practice 95
Unit 13   Communicating Evidence: Critical Conversations 107

Appendix 113
Master List of Worksheets by Unit 114
References in Alphabetical Order 149
References by Unit 153
Index. 159

Instructors: *Bringing Evidence Into Everyday Practice: Practical Strategies for Health Care Professionals,
Second Edition,* includes ancillary materials specifically available for faculty use. Included is an
Instructor's Manual. Please visit www.routledge.com/9781638220695 to obtain access.

MASTER LIST OF WORKSHEETS

The Appendix contains a reference list and accompanying grid of these worksheets by unit, showing which worksheets will be used in each unit. Instructors can access and download fillable PDFs of the worksheets at www.routledge.com/9781638220695

Analyze and Improve the Precision of Participant Criteria 116
Analyze Intervention Practices to Determine Whether They Are Controversial 117
Analyze the Results Section of an Article 118
Apply Evidence to a Specific Situation 119
Compare and Contrast Take-Home Messages 120
Compare Evidence Classification Systems 121
Compare Intervention Programs 122
Create a Rationale for Summary Points From an Article 123
Create Take-Home Messages 124
Examine the Similarities and Differences in the Summary Tables 125
Examine Ways to Expand Knowledge About Assistive Devices 126
Find Similarities in Conceptual Themes 127
Find Unique Themes Across Studies 128
Identify Answerable and Unanswerable Questions 129
Identify Familiar Research Concepts 130
Identify New Research Concepts 131
Identify Search Parameters in a Summary Study 132
Integrate Data About Smart Devices From a Systematic Review 133
List Evidence-Based Practice Concepts 134
List Steps in Implementing Evidence-Based Practice 135
Look for Themes Across Studies: Part 1 136
Look for Themes Across Studies: Part 2 137
Progress Monitoring Plan 138
Reactions to New Data 139
Review the Parts of a Research Article 140
Summarize Intervention Studies 141
Summarize Key Points for Analysis 142
Summarize the Characteristics of a Research Article 143
Summarize the Inclusion Criteria 144
Summarize Themes in the Introduction 145
Summary Table for Sensory Processing Patterns 146
Write Brief Take-Home Messages 147
Your Response to Others' Reactions to New Data 148

Worksheet	Unit												
	1	2	3	4	5	6	7	8	9	10	11	12	13
Analyze and Improve			X										
Analyze Intervention											X		
Analyze the Results									X				
Apply Evidence										X			
Compare and Contrast													X
Compare Evidence	X												
Compare Intervention								X					
Create a Rationale							X						
Create Take-Home Messages			X	X	X	X	X	X	X	X	X		X
Examine the Similarities			X										
Examine Ways				X									
Find Similarities						X							
Find Unique Themes						X							
Identify Answerable			X	X	X	X	X	X	X				
Identify Familiar	X												
Identify New	X												
Identify Search										X			
Integrate Data				X									
List Evidence-Based	X												
List Steps	X												
Look for Themes 1					X								
Look for Themes 2					X								
Progress Monitoring Plan												X	
Reactions to New Data		X	X	X	X	X	X	X	X	X	X		X
Review the Parts			X										
Summarize Intervention			X										
Summarize Key Points											X		
Summarize the Characteristics			X	X	X	X	X	X	X		X		
Summarize the Inclusion			X										
Summarize Themes			X										
Summary Table							X						
Write Brief			X										
Your Response		X											X

ACKNOWLEDGMENTS

This book is a departure from the traditional textbooks on the market; it took vision and tenacity from the publisher to move this project into the marketplace. We are grateful to Brien Cummings for his trust in creating a contemporary version of this workbook.

It was also a complex task to gather the materials and select what would be the best learning options for students and colleagues. We are grateful to Angie Williams for her overall support and Kasten Colvin for steady focus on the details of each unit.

Material for a workbook requires tryouts to make sure that the activities are understandable and useful to professionals in practice. We acknowledge all the providers who have learned about and studied evidence-based practices with us—you showed us what matters. We also acknowledge all the graduate students who have studied this topic with us; you asked many questions that invited us to understand better, and therefore teach better.

ABOUT THE AUTHORS

Winnie Dunn, PhD, OTR, FAOTA, is a Distinguished Professor in the Department of Occupational Therapy Education at the University of Missouri and is a Certified Positive Psychology Coach. She was the Eleanor Clarke Slagle lecturer in 2001, received the Award of Merit from the American Occupational Therapy Association, received the A. Jean Ayres research award and the Chancellor's teaching and research awards, served as a Kemper Teaching Fellow, and is a member of the Academy of Research of the American Occupational Therapy Foundation. She has contributed research and other writings to professional literature across her career. Currently she is studying the impact of evidence-based coaching practices on family, education, and child outcomes.

Believing that researchers must also translate their findings for the public, she has also published her book *Living Sensationally: Understanding Your Senses,* which is available in several languages. Its focus is to demonstrate how sensory processing is part of everyone's choices throughout their daily routines. The book is written in everyday language so that everyone can understand their own, their family's, their coworkers', and their friends' behaviors a little better.

Rachel Proffitt, OTD, OTR/L, is an Associate Professor in the Department of Occupational Therapy at the University of Missouri. She received her OTD from Washington University in St. Louis and completed a T32 post-doctoral fellowship at the University of Southern California. She has a Certificate in Clinical, Translational, and Biomedical Investigations and was awarded the ASA/ACRM Young Investigator Award in Post-Acute Stroke Rehabilitation in 2020. Her research spans the breadth of technology, including virtual reality and ambient sensors to support individuals post-stroke and older adults living in the community. She has received foundation and federal funding to support her research, including an Intervention Research Grant from the American Occupational Therapy Foundation. She is the principal investigator of a 3-year R01 exploring a technology-supported intervention for rural community–dwelling older adults with disabilities.

PREFACE

I just love workbooks! I have loved them all my life. When I was a girl, I would work my way through the puzzle books and the little scratch pads with notes to myself as I worked. My favorite games were "Who drinks milk?" and "Who owns the zebra?" These are the logic games that provide you with a set of statements like "The family in the green house likes to drink milk; they live next to the family that owns a zebra." You had to create a grid that had every family's house color, pet, drink, car type, and number of members from all these statements. Whew! They were challenging, but boy did I get some brain aerobics from them.

So, as I have worked through problems in our profession, this idea of figuring out the puzzle always comes to mind. At first it was me and an article, trying to decipher what the table told me, what the text meant, or figure out what the graph illustrated. As I began to teach, I had to construct methods for introducing this problem solving to others. This workbook is a selection of my puzzles and their solutions, I hope they are as helpful to you as they have been for me and others.

And now I have a partner in finding solutions! Rachel Proffitt is a colleague who shares this passion for digging in to find solutions, and for supporting others to find their own ways of finding meaning in the research process. It makes me so happy to see this legacy of having fun while thinking deeply continue through the next generations of professionals.

The workbook is in three sections. In the first section, we explore the basic ideas of evidence and research for practice. In the second section, you get a chance to practice with topics that will inform various areas of practice; we use the same general format in each unit, so you can apply that format to other groups of articles that are interesting to you. In the third section, we delve into some advanced ideas about evidence in practice, so you have even more tools at your disposal.

Enjoy our professional puzzle book!

—*Winnie Dunn, PhD, OTR, FAOTA*

INTRODUCTION

Professionals are increasingly being asked to base their decisions on evidence. We all agree that this is a good idea, no one wants to spend precious time engaging in strategies that are not likely to be effective. Systematic reviews of the literature provide one excellent resource, because scholars summarize a body of literature about a topic for the field. However, there is not a large body of literature to support all the things we encounter in everyday practice.

With the internet readily available, professionals can search for literature on topics of interest to their practice. But just having found some articles doesn't ensure evidence-based practice either. Professionals must know how to mine the gold from these sources to make informed decisions for their everyday practice. With time at a premium, professionals need specific and efficient strategies for using the literature to craft evidence-based plans for their practice.

This book provides the strategies for translating evidence into everyday practice. It provides the initial steps that a single professional, an interdisciplinary team, or a study group can use to build solid decision-making patterns that will support their practices. This is not a book for scholarly review of the literature; scholars have resources for this task and are increasingly providing us with excellent material we can use on topics with a wealth of information available.

There are textbooks that discuss more formal ways to review the literature (e.g., Law & MacDermid, 2014). There are other texts that will guide you through the research design and statistics used to support research; we will discuss these issues as they arise within an article of interest (e.g., Brown, 2016; Portney, 2020). Use one of these texts, or your own design and statistics text, to learn more about a study's features.

Instead, this book will help professionals entering practice or in practice to take the first steps toward including evidence in their everyday decisions. We will examine how to access meta-analyses or systematic reviews, but we will also examine how to evaluate the two to three articles a team finds that address the dilemma they are facing that week in their service system. As professionals gain more confidence about how to access and use the literature on a small scale, the concept of evidence-based practice will feel more attainable for everyone.

Resource Book on Evidence-Based Practice for This Book

Law, M., & MacDermid, J. (2014). Evidence-based rehabilitation: A guide to practice (3rd ed.). SLACK Incorporated. ISBN-10: 1617110213, ISBN-13: 9781617110214.

This book is an excellent reference to help you understand the concepts of evidence-based practice. The authors provide many good examples of how professionals formally analyze the literature to determine what best practices ought to be.

Other Recommended Resources That Address Research Design and Statistics

Portney, L. G. (Ed.). (2020). Foundations of clinical research: Applications to evidence-based practice *(4th ed.). F. A. Davis Company. ISBN-10: 0803661134, ISBN-13: 9780803661134, https:// fadavispt.mhmedical.com/*

This book is an excellent reference to help you understand research designs, methods, statistical procedures, and results in research articles. As you read articles, use this text to understand the methods and results that the authors describe.

Brown, C. (2016). The evidence-based practitioner: Applying research to meet client needs *(2nd ed.). F. A. Davis Company. ISBN-10: 1719642818, ISBN-13: 9781719642811.*

This book is also an excellent reference to support your learning about research designs and statistical procedures. This text can serve as a reference when you don't understand something in an article you are reading.

Overview of This Book

The book is divided into three sections. Section I introduces the reader to basic evidence-based practice concepts. Section II provides opportunities for practicing how to gather information and summarize it for use in practice. Section III addresses additional issues in evidence-based practice.

Section I: Learning the Basics

Section I contains basic information about evidence-based practice principles and methods.

Unit 1

Introduction to the Concepts of Evidence-Based Practice

During this unit, you will explore the general concepts of evidence-based practice and research. You will review articles that discuss the core concepts and issues of evidence-based practice, read about research as a resource for professional practice, have a discussion with your study partners about what you learned, find a newer article that adds to your discussion, and share it with your study partners.

Searching Databases

There is a wealth of information available to professionals, but one needs to know how to gain access to this relevant material. In this unit, you will explore professional databases and learn how to access relevant information effectively and efficiently.

Determining the Quality of the Evidence

Some studies provide stronger evidence than other studies because of how they were designed. You will learn some of the classification systems that enable you to know the level of a study's contribution to your knowledge for evidence-based practice.

Unit 2

Handling Anomalous Data

Another really important issue to address when working to create an evidence-based practice is how you personally react to ideas that come your way. It is human nature to be attracted to information that agrees with your beliefs and to be skeptical about information that challenges your beliefs. We will learn a framework for understanding reactions to new ideas in practice during this unit.

Unit 3

Basic Characteristics of Research Articles

It is hard to be evidence-based professionals without some understanding of how research articles are constructed. Professionals can expect to obtain certain information from different parts of the research article; these expectations serve as guideposts for evidence-based practice. You can compare the population you serve to the study group, you can decide whether the measures in the study document behaviors that matter to you, and you can determine whether the intervention itself might be manageable for your practice. In this unit, you will explore the parts of a research article so you can be a better evidence-based professional.

Practice With an Entire Article

We will walk through an article together, studying the details of its structure, creating hypotheses along with the authors, and practicing writing interpretations in your own words.

Section II: Practice Using Evidence to Design Best Practices

It takes practice to learn how to uncover the evidence. In this section you will practice analyzing research articles. You will learn many strategies that you can use in your professional practice. We will cover the following topics in our evidence-based reviews (Units 4 through 9):

- Evidence about the use of assistive devices with older adults and people with disabilities
- Evidence about the use of compensatory strategies with community-dwelling adults who have schizophrenia
- Evidence about caregiving across the life span
- Evidence about sensory profiles for children across stages of development
- Evidence about the use of constraint-induced therapy with persons who have had a stroke
- Evidence about therapy for upper extremity fractures in adults and children

There are many other topics we could cover, but this gives you a range of topics to get you started.

Section III: Expanding Your Knowledge and Skills for Evidence-Based Practice

There are additional resources available to support evidence-based practice. Scholars conduct formal reviews of the literature so you can have summaries and recommendations from others. Emerging ideas in professional practice often don't have evidence, so you need to have other strategies for evaluating these ideas. Professionals also need to collect their own data within their practices to verify the effectiveness of any evidence, emerging or established. Lastly, communicating evidence to consumers and stakeholders is an important component of the evidence-based practice triad. We will review these topics in Section III.

Unit 10

Summary and Meta-Analysis Articles

Scholars review sets of articles and provide a summary of the findings in both summary and meta-analysis articles. This is a great resource for professionals who have very little time to conduct exhaustive reviews. You will learn how to read and take advantage of these resources.

Unit 11

Examining Emerging and Controversial Practices

What do professionals do with new ideas? How do we determine whether a new idea is worthy of our attention as evidence-based professionals? This unit will introduce you to some strategies for analyzing new or controversial ideas so you can incorporate promising interventions and set aside other ideas from your practice.

Unit 12

Developing Evidence for Your Own Practice

No matter how much evidence is available, professionals still don't know whether an intervention will work in **their** practices. Collecting data within professional practice provides validity that the intervention is effective with that person in that situation. We can also try out an intervention not typically used in a population by collecting data to determine the appropriateness of the generalization.

Unit 13

Communicating Evidence

How does your client know that the intervention you have chosen will work for them? What if you want to try a new protocol or program in your practice setting and your manager is resistant to change? These critical conversations are a key part of the evidence-based practice process. You will have opportunities to practice with your peers and instructor. The scripts you create will provide a framework for future conversations in practice.

How to Use This Book

This book will take you step-by-step to learn how to incorporate evidence into your everyday practice. Please read the bulleted list on page xxiii to learn about the different components used throughout this book to help you with this process.

Summary

Many texts provide academic knowledge about evidence-based practice, this book will give you the tools to implement sound ideas in your professional life.

HOW TO USE THIS BOOK

The goal of this book is to help readers learn how to incorporate evidence into their everyday decisions. The book contains several different elements to help achieve this goal.

- Each unit contains activities that assist readers, step by step, toward incorporating evidence into everyday decisions.
- Throughout the book we ask readers to read certain journal articles that will be used as the basis for the unit activities and worksheets. The text provides the bibliographic information of each article, including the DOI (digital object identifier), so that readers can locate the article online within their own library systems.
- Each unit refers to worksheets to structure the reader's practice and learning. Instructors can access fillable PDFs of these worksheets at www.routledge.com/ 9781638220695 The Appendix contains the Master List of Worksheets by Unit and accompanying grid, with reference to when they are needed within the units.
- Sidebars include important material to assist in learning, performing the activities, and completing the worksheets. The sidebars are referenced in the text.
- "Evidence Detective Tips" give readers additional helpful hints regarding research studies and practice.
- An alphabetical bibliography begins on page 149; a bibliography by unit begins on page 153.

Online Materials

The online materials supplement the physical textbook. There are several components to assist both learners and instructors.

- Fillable PDFs of all of worksheets found in the book.
- Many of the worksheets are used in multiple chapters. The Master List of Worksheets by Unit and accompanying grid shows which worksheet is used in which unit.
- The online bibliography of all articles used in the book includes the DOI link to the article at the journal website.
- The *Instructor's Manual* includes several components:
  - A mapping of the textbook activities with the book *Effective Teaching: Instructional Methods and Strategies for Occupational Therapy Education* by Dr. Whitney Henderson. Instructors can customize activities using evidence-based teaching strategies.
  - A mapping of the units to the resource textbooks (Brown, 2016; Law & MacDermid, 2014; Portney, 2020). This can be helpful in assigning pre-class readings.
  - Sample plans for each unit, including preparatory, in-class, and homework activities.
  - Instructor notes for some units that require more in-depth discussion of topics.
  - A sample syllabus and semester schedule.

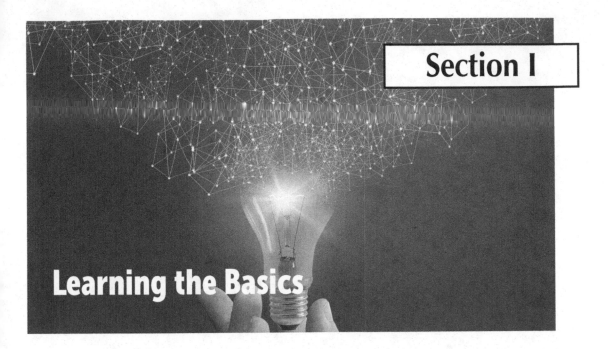

Section I

Learning the Basics

BACKGROUND KNOWLEDGE FOR
EVIDENCE-BASED PRACTICE

In the first section of this manual, you will explore the basic concepts of evidence-based practice, examine your own patterns of accepting or rejecting evidence that challenges your current beliefs, and learn how to look at the Methods and Results sections of professional articles.

Introduction to Evidence-Based Practice

During this unit, we will explore the general concepts of evidence-based practice. You will review articles and participate in discussions with classmates or colleagues about the concepts of evidence-based practice. You will also find a newer article that informs this discussion and share the abstract with your classmates/colleagues (your study partners).

When you complete the work for this unit, you will have the following skills and competencies:

- Identifying what you already know about basic research concepts
- Identifying new concepts you need to know about research
- Becoming familiar with evidence-based practice language
- Recognizing interdisciplinary issues in evidence-based practice
- Articulating the importance of evidence-based practice
- Identifying initial strategies for implementing evidence-based practice in your practice
- Understanding how to select key words for searching in library databases
- Identifying advanced search strategies to obtain critical information
- Sorting through possible citations to identify relevant ones
- Becoming familiar with the levels of evidence

Dunn, W., & Proffitt, R. *Bringing Evidence Into Everyday Practice: Practical Strategies for Health Care Professionals, Second Edition* (pp. 3-8).
© 2024 Taylor & Francis Group.

IDENTIFY WHAT YOU ALREADY KNOW AND IDENTIFY NEW CONCEPTS ENCOUNTERED

Research studies that demonstrate the effectiveness or limitations of particular strategies provide the material for evidence-based practice. Professionals need to have a basic understanding about research concepts so they can decide whether the research they are reading is worthy of consideration. You will notice that you are familiar with some of the material as your read about research concepts, while other concepts will be new to you.

Activity 1-1
Read the Literature

Worksheet: Identify Familiar Research Concepts
Worksheet: Identify New Research Concepts

Read a chapter about research from your own research design textbook (or you can read Chapter 1 in Portney [2020] or Chapter 1 in Brown [2016]).

Complete these worksheets to summarize what is familiar and new to you. There is an example at the beginning of each worksheet.

Activity 1-2
Discuss

Meet with study partners and discuss what each of you learned about research concepts. If you have examples of these concepts being used in a study you have read, bring this to share with your study partners.

FAMILIARIZE YOURSELF WITH EVIDENCE-BASED PRACTICE LANGUAGE

Knowledge about research concepts is necessary, but insufficient for evidence-based practice. Professionals must also know the language and structure for employing evidence-based practices. We must understand what people mean when they say "evidence-based practice" so we can meet the expectations within our work. Law and MacDermid (2014) provide an excellent summary about evidence-based practice to guide your thinking.

Activity 1-3
Consider Applications

Worksheet: List Evidence-Based Practice Concepts

Read Chapters 1 through 3 in Law and MacDermid (2014). These chapters provide a good background for understanding evidence-based practice. Think about how these ideas might relate to your areas of practice interest and brainstorm ideas about applications in practice with your study partners. Complete the worksheet to summarize your thoughts.

We can obtain information about evidence-based practice from journal articles as well as textbooks. Sometimes articles are helpful because they focus on one aspect of evidence-based practice, enabling the reader to tailor work on an aspect of interest to the reader's practice.

Activity 1-4
Read and Discuss

Worksheet: List Steps in Implementing Evidence-Based Practice

Obtain and read the five articles listed here. They discuss the five steps in implementing evidence-based practice (using the worksheet). You will see that these articles are older than we would typically recommend as contemporary resources. We continue to use them because they are succinct summaries of the key elements of evidence-based practice that are still applicable today and therefore are great resources for new learners.

Tickle-Degnen, L. (1999). Evidence-based practice forum. Organizing, evaluating, and using evidence. American Journal of Occupational Therapy, 53(6), 537-539. https://doi.org/10.5014/ajot.53.5.537

Tickle-Degnen, L. (2000a). Evidence-based practice forum. Communicating with clients, family members, and colleagues about research evidence. American Journal of Occupational Therapy, 54(3), 341-343. https://doi.org/10.5014/ajot.54.3.341

Tickle-Degnen, L. (2000b). Evidence-based practice forum. Gathering current research evidence to enhance clinical reasoning. American Journal of Occupational Therapy, 54(1), 102-105. https://doi.org/10.5014/ajot.54.1.102

Tickle-Degnen, L. (2000c). Evidence-based practice forum. Monitoring and documenting evidence during assessment and intervention. American Journal of Occupational Therapy, 54(4), 434-436. https://doi.org/10.5014/ajot.54.4.434

Tickle-Degnen, L. (2000d). Evidence-based practice forum. What is the best evidence to use in practice? American Journal of Occupational Therapy, 54(2), 218-221. https://doi.org/10.5014/ajot.54.2.218

Activity 1-5
Select and Reflect

Select one additional article on evidence-based practice that is applicable to your interests.

Bannigan, K., & Moores, A. (2009). *A model of professional thinking: Integrating reflective practice and evidence-based practice.* Canadian Journal of Occupational Therapy, 76(5), 342-350. https://doi.org/10.1177%2F000841740907600505

Dirette, D., Rozich, A., & Viau, S. (2009). *Is there enough evidence for evidence-based practice in occupational therapy?* American Journal of Occupational Therapy, 63(6), 782-786. https://doi.org/10.5014/ajot.63.6.782

Ilott, I. (2003). *Evidence-based practice forum. Challenging the rhetoric and reality: Only an individual and systemic approach will work for evidence-based occupational therapy.* American Journal of Occupational Therapy, 57(3), 351-354. https://doi.org/10.5014/ajot.57.3.351

Lee, C. J., & Miller, L. T. (2003). *Evidence-based practice forum. The process of evidence-based clinical decision making in occupational therapy.* American Journal of Occupational Therapy, 57(4), 473-477. https://doi.org/10.5014/ajot.57.4.473

Ottenbacher, K. J., Tickle-Degnen, L., & Hasselkus, B. R. (2002). *From the desk of the editor. Therapists awake! The challenge of evidence-based occupational therapy.* American Journal of Occupational Therapy, 56(3), 247-249. https://doi.org/10.5014/ajot.56.3.247

Rappolt, S. (2003). *Evidence-based practice forum. The role of professional expertise in evidence-based occupational therapy.* American Journal of Occupational Therapy, 57(5), 589-593. https://doi.org/10.5014/ajot.57.5.589

Thomas, A., & Law, M. (2013). *Research utilization and evidence-based practice in occupational therapy: A scoping study.* American Journal of Occupational Therapy, 67(4), e55-e65. https://doi.org/10.5014/ajot.2013.006395

Tickle-Degnen, L. (2003). *Evidence-based practice forum. Where is the individual in statistics?* American Journal of Occupational Therapy, 57(1), 112-115. https://doi.org/10.5014/ajot.57.1.112

Tickle-Degnen, L., & Bedell, G. (2003). *Evidence-based practice forum. Heterarchy and hierarchy: A critical appraisal of the levels of evidence as a tool for clinical decision making.* American Journal of Occupational Therapy, 57(2), 234-237. https://doi.org/10.5014/ajot.57.2.234

EVIDENCE-BASED PRACTICE IS AN INTERDISCIPLINARY ISSUE

No matter what professional background one has, the call for evidence-based practice is strong. Some disciplines have been working on these issues for a long time, while other disciplines are just starting to consider how to incorporate evidence in their practices. Since we all work on interdisciplinary teams, it is important to know how other disciplines are dealing with similar issues.

Activity 1-6
Compare and Contrast

Locate an article about evidence-based practice from another discipline. Read the article and consider similarities and differences from your own discipline. Consider whether this other discipline has ideas that might be useful to your thinking as you plan to implement evidence-based practices.

For this activity, you can use "evidence-based practice" as one of your search phrases. Add to it the name of another discipline (e.g., "nursing"). The search engine will select only articles with both these concepts in them. You could also add "children" and you would get only articles about children, nursing, and evidence-based practice. Some search engines let you select where to search; you might want to limit the search to the titles, abstract, and key words (rather than the whole article) so you narrow your list to only those articles that use the search words in these sections of the article.

Activity 1-7
Discuss

Meet with study partners.
- Discuss what additional information you gained from reading the articles (Activities 1-4 and 1-5).
- Did the articles give you more ideas about how to implement evidence-based practice in your areas of interest?
- Discuss ideas you obtained from reading an interdisciplinary article (Activity 1-6).
- How could this discipline's perspective contribute to your thinking?

SEARCH PROFESSIONAL DATABASES
TO FIND ARTICLES

Professionals need to know how to conduct searches using various search engines and databases. Most professional libraries have learning modules prepared by the librarians to teach you about conducting a search. You can also access these experts to help you in person. If you are inexperienced at using search strategies, you can also take a class at a library, use the Help section of your search engine (e.g., MEDLINE, CINAHL), or try out some strategies on Google Scholar (it has a section on tips for searching).

Chapter 5 of the Law and MacDermid (2014) text also explains how to search in the literature.

Activity 1-8
Practice Searching in Professional Databases

Select a professional database that is relevant to your area of interest. Put in one key word and see how many references you get. Add one or two more words to your list and see how these key words narrow your list. Then go back to your original word and enter two different key words. Compare the two lists. Sometimes narrowing with certain key words makes your list more precise; narrowing can also divert your list away from your specific interest areas.

If you know an author who is an expert in an area, you can also search by that person's name along with key words.

DETERMINE THE QUALITY OF EVIDENCE

In addition to understanding how to look at the parts of a research article, professionals are responsible for considering the quality of the studies. This is because quality helps you to know how much influence the findings need to have in your practice.

Chapter 6 in Law and MacDermid (2014) provides a summary of various methods that researchers use to determine the level of evidence that a particular study contributes to knowledge. There are other classifications systems available. Many are specific to a health care profession or a specialized area of practice.

Activity 1-9
Compare and Contrast

Worksheet: Compare Evidence Classification Systems

Using the classification systems listed here, complete a comparison of the similarities and differences between the three systems. Discuss the advantages and disadvantages with your study partners.

What are the advantages and disadvantages of these approaches? Discuss which classification system is most useful for your work. As we encounter articles in this manual and in your practice, consider the levels of evidence each article represents to your knowledge.

Although it is important for you to be aware that many classification systems exist, your faculty member may ask you to use one of these classification systems for an assignment in class to provide you with some practice. Here are some resources for you:

Balshem, H., Helfand, M., Schuneman, H. J., Oxman, A. D., Kunz, R., Brozek, J., Vist, G., Falck-Ytter, Y., Meerpohl, J., Norris, S., & Guyatt, G. H. (2011). GRADE guidelines: 3. Rating the quality of evidence. Journal of Clinical Epidemiology, 64, 401-406. https://doi.org/10.1016/j.jclinepi.2010.07.015

OCEBM Levels of Evidence Working Group*. (n.d.). The Oxford Levels of Evidence 2. Oxford Centre for Evidence-Based Medicine. https://www.cebm.ox.ac.uk/resources/levels-of-evidence/ocebm-levels-of-evidence

Tomlin, G., & Borgetto, B. (2011). Research pyramid: A new evidence-based practice model for occupational therapy. American Journal of Occupational Therapy, 65(2), 189-196. https://doi.org/10.5014/ajot.2011.000828

SUMMARY

This unit introduced you to concepts that form the basis for evidence-based practice. Mastering these concepts and skills enables you to understand the evidence you will encounter in your practice.

Characterizing Responses to Evidence

When professionals encounter evidence that may affect their practices, they must decide what they are going to do with that information. Sometimes research isn't relevant to a particular situation. Research projects may be done poorly and, therefore, have to be set aside. Research may support a professional's current practices; these studies are easy to embrace. Research may also be relevant to one's practice, but findings may challenge what the professional currently believes to be true. As evidence-based practitioners, professionals need to understand how to handle these various scenarios.

It is human nature to be attracted to information that agrees with our beliefs and to be skeptical about information that challenges our beliefs. However, as professionals, we have a responsibility to remain open to new possibilities. Across one's career it is easy to see that ideas progress, and what is considered acceptable practice changes as we understand more. But individually and as a team, it can be easy to get stuck in protocols or routines that were originally based on best available knowledge but become outdated as new information becomes available. We have to acknowledge that this sometimes happens, and we have to push ourselves to consider alternatives every day of our professional careers.

Sometimes it is appropriate and necessary to reject or ignore data. Evidence-based practice does not mean professionals accept every new piece of information that comes along. Using evidence in practice does mean that professionals critically analyze their reactions to make sure that new information is given proper consideration.

When you complete the work for this unit, you will have the following skills and competencies:

- Understanding the different ways people respond to new or challenging data
- Recognizing different ways people will react and what their reactions mean
- Formulating a strategy for analyzing your own responses to new or challenging data in your practice

Dunn, W., & Proffitt, R. *Bringing Evidence Into Everyday Practice: Practical Strategies for Health Care Professionals, Second Edition* (pp. 9-12).
© 2024 Taylor & Francis Group.

WAYS TO HANDLE ANOMALOUS DATA

There is an older article from the education literature that provides some structure for considering alternatives for handling new or unfamiliar data. In 1993, Chinn and Brewer wrote an article about how children learn science. Their ideas extend well beyond this initial goal and provide a wonderful framework for considering our reactions to new and potentially challenging information. They discuss "anomalous data" as "evidence that contradicts a person's current theories about how something happens/works."

Chinn and Brewer (1993) propose that people respond in seven possible ways when presented with anomalous data (Sidebar 2-1). Let's review the seven different ways people respond. Think of times you have responded in each of these seven ways.

Activity 2-1
Read the Literature

Worksheet: Reactions to New Data

Read the Chinn and Brewer (1993) excerpt (pp. 1-49):

Chinn, C. A., & Brewer, W. F. (1993). *The role of anomalous data in knowledge acquisition: A theoretical framework and implications for science instruction.* Review of Educational Research, *63(1), 1-49. https://doi.org/10.3102/00346543063001001*

Take note of the seven ways that people respond to new or challenging information. Think of a situation in practice that would illustrate each of the seven patterns. Complete the worksheet to record your thoughts. Sidebar 2-1 provides an executive summary for you.

Activity 2-2
Discuss

Worksheet: Your Response to Others' Reactions to New Data

Meet with your study partners and be prepared to discuss Terrance's case (Sidebar 2-2) based on what you learned from the Chinn and Brewer (1993) article. Write a scenario for each of Chinn and Brewer's (1993) responses that would illustrate Terrance's response to this new information.

Sidebar 2-1
Executive Summary of Chinn and Brewer (1993)

Anomalous Data

This article presents a detailed analysis of the ways in which scientists and science students respond to [anomalous] data. We postulate that there are seven distinct forms of response. One is to accept the data, and the other six responses involve discounting the data in various ways (p. 1).

Anomalous data: Evidence that contradicts a person's current theories about how something happens/works.

Seven Possible Responses to Anomalous Data

1. **IGNORE** the anomalous data. People ignore data when the data are contradictory to their view about how things work. They don't even bother to explain why the data are contrary when they are ignoring it.

   Look for examples where the professional demonstrates lack of interest in the topic, perhaps not seeing the relevance of a particular area of writing for the professional's practice areas.

2. **REJECT** the anomalous data. People also reject data when they are contradictory to their current views. The unique feature of rejection is that the person will explain why data should be rejected.

   Look for examples in which the professional provides a justification for rejecting particular information. A therapist might reject findings from an article because measures were weak, there weren't enough participants, or that it was the ONLY study in the area of interest.

3. **EXCLUDE** the anomalous data. People exclude data by deciding that the data reveal information that is relevant for some other discipline or area of expertise, but not their own.

   Look for explanations about why particular information doesn't apply to the current practices and beliefs. A therapist might exclude data about spasticity because the study is about children and the therapist serves adults.

4. Hold the anomalous data in **ABEYANCE**. People hold the data in abeyance by delaying their willingness to deal with the data. They continue to hold their current beliefs and acknowledge that someday the ideas in the data will be articulated so that it will change current beliefs.

   Look for explanations that focus on current beliefs and how they are not developed enough to account for the new finding. A therapist might hold data showing that traditional neurodevelopmental treatment (NDT) doesn't work in abeyance by saying that there aren't good enough measures yet.

5. **REINTERPRET** the anomalous data. People reinterpret the data by formulating an explanation about the data that is consistent with their current beliefs, even though the researchers have articulated a different explanation for the findings.

   Look for explanations that show two different explanations for the same findings. An occupational therapist thinks that the findings show the power of sensory processing, while the behaviorist thinks that the findings show the power of contingencies.

6. **MAKE PERIPHERAL CHANGES** in the theory. People make peripheral changes to their current beliefs by making a minor change to their current beliefs, but retaining the core of their current ideas.

   Look for explanations that compartmentalize the findings into one small part. The therapist says that recovery models might be OK for some mental health disorders, but not the ones that they work with.

7. Accept the data and **CHANGE** the theory. People accept data by changing a core belief based on data (as we might do as we begin to implement evidence-based practice).

   Look for explanations that show a shift in a belief within the practice. The therapist decides that the team needs to stop doing range of motion exercises because studies have shown they don't contribute to the functional outcomes they desire.

Parts reproduced with permission from Chinn, C. A., & Brewer, W. F. (1993). The role of anomalous data in knowledge acquisition: A theoretical framework and implications for science instruction. *Review of Educational Research, 63*(1), 1-49.

Sidebar 2-2
Case Study: Terrance

Terrance has been working in a rehabilitation setting for 10 years. He is proud of his work. He focuses on retraining activities of daily living (ADLs) in the early part of rehabilitation and works on functional supports for the individual and their family as part of transition planning.

Terrance is part of a study group. Last week they read an article about Cognitive Orientation to daily Occupational Performance (CO-OP). CO-OP teaches clients a global problem-solving approach that can be generalized to novel activities and contexts: Goal-Plan-Do-Check. The study group had a lively discussion. Now Terrance is faced with having to consider whether he needs to change his rehabilitation practices.

SUMMARY

Understanding reactions to new information is a critical part of evidence-based practice. Sometimes reactions to reject or hold data in abeyance are appropriate, and other times these reactions represent fear or reluctance to think a new way. Considering all possibilities enables professionals to understand themselves, their colleagues, and the people they serve a little better. Critical analyses of one's reactions to new data ensure that the best possible professional practices are being implemented.

Understanding and Using the Basic Parts of Research Articles

In this unit, you will explore some of the basic parts of research articles. When you understand the parts of a research article, you will know where to look for the information you need to apply evidence in your practice.

When researchers set out, there are some conventions everyone follows to report the findings. Each professional journal has a stylized way of presenting the information, but the same basic information is available no matter what style journals select. Portney (2020) provides a summary of the parts of research articles in Chapter 36, "Critical Appraisal: Evaluating Research Reports"—use this reference as a guide to your learning.

When you complete the work for this unit, you will have the following skills and competencies:

- Identifying the key sections of a research article
- Summarizing what you will find in each section of a research article
- Recognizing the strengths and weaknesses of operational definitions in an article
- Deriving meaning from the Results section of an article
- Reading and interpret tables and figures in articles
- Linking research questions, methods, results, and discussion

Keep your research design and statistics reference books handy; when you are reviewing an article, look up the design and statistical analyses the authors are using. These texts typically do a great job of explaining what these procedures mean and how to interpret them for your practice. By doing this every time you review an article, you will build your repertoire of background knowledge.

Dunn, W., & Proffitt, R. *Bringing Evidence Into Everyday Practice: Practical Strategies for Health Care Professionals, Second Edition* (pp. 13-26). © 2024 Taylor & Francis Group.

Activity 3-1
Read the Literature

Read Chapter 4 in the Law and MacDermid (2014) text to provide you with some background about research articles. Focus on the sections that discuss how to measure outcomes, including the discussion about statistical outcomes. Jot down notes about key points that will help you when you read articles.

Activity 3-2
Read the Literature

Read the chapter in your research design text that provides an overview of the parts of research articles and guidance about what to ask yourself as you read articles (e.g., Section 3 of Portney, 2020).

BASIC SECTIONS OF RESEARCH ARTICLES

Traditionally there are five parts to a research article. The Title and Abstract provide the reader with an overview of the work that will be reported. You can decide whether you are interested in the article by looking at this summary. Because the Title and Abstract are brief, the reader cannot determine the strength of the study or its applicability to certain practice situations from just this part of an article.

The Introduction provides background about the subject matter and builds a case for this study. The reader can get familiarized with relevant literature and understand what gaps there may be, which creates the need for the study to be reported. Toward the end of the Introduction, the authors provide the research questions, hypotheses, or problem statements that frame the current study's work.

The Methods section provides the reader with the blueprint for the study. All the essential elements about who, what, where, when, and how must be reported here. There should also be enough detail that the reader can imagine all parts of the study and another researcher could conduct a similar study.

Because the Methods section provides details about the study structure, there are several sections. The *Participants* section describes who the authors will study. The *Design* section explains how the study is organized. The *Instrumentation* section describes what measures are used in the study. The *Procedures* section explains the sequence of events to complete the study. The *Data Analysis* section describes how data were analyzed to determine the outcomes.

The Results section provides the reader with the findings of the study. The reader should expect only facts in this section of a research article. The reader should expect to see tables and figures summarizing findings. The authors must report on each hypothesis or research question in the Results section.

Interpretive material is reserved for the Discussion section. This is the place for the author to reflect on the findings of the study and provide the reader with the author's insights about the meaning of the study findings. Many times, authors will link their findings to literature, pointing out both similarities and differences with the current study.

Activity 3-3
Practice With an Article

Worksheet: Review the Parts of a Research Article

Read the following article:

Schwandt, M., Harris, J. E., Thomas, S., Keightley, M., Snaiderman, A., & Colantonio, A. (2012). *Feasibility and effect of aerobic exercise for lowering depressive symptoms among individuals with traumatic brain injury: A pilot study.* Journal of Head Trauma Rehabilitation, *27(2), 99-103.* https://doi.org/10.1097/HTR.0b013e31820e6858

Complete the worksheet as you review the Schwandt et al. (2012) article. Observe how your ideas change as you move from the Abstract to the Introduction.

- As you read the Methods section, take note of the new considerations that occur to you.
- Do your reactions change when you encounter the results?
- Do the authors change your perspective with their insights in the Discussion?

PRACTICE EXAMINING PARTICIPANT CRITERIA (METHODS SECTION)

Now that you have some initial practice, let's look at some of the parts of research articles by themselves. For example, by looking at the details of the Methods sections, we learn whether the articles relate to specific populations or can be generalized. We also learn whether the researchers designed the studies properly. This activity will increase your discrimination ability when engaging in evidence-based practice.

One of the important details is the participant population. This section of the Methods enables you to decide if a study is applicable to your practice. Specifically, researchers provide details about who they will include and exclude in their study. Read the inclusion and exclusion criteria in the worksheet. Then, consider how you would implement these criteria to select participants.

Activity 3-4
Learn About Inclusion and Exclusion Criteria

Worksheet: Analyze and Improve the Precision of Participant Criteria

You can see from this list of criteria (in Column 1 of the worksheet) that it is not perfectly clear who would be included or excluded from the participant pool. For example, what criteria would be used to decide whether someone is "able to communicate and follow verbal instructions in English"? Use the worksheet to identify what questions you have about these criteria, and then write an improved version of the criteria. For example, what would you observe or what test score would you use to decide whether someone was "able to follow verbal instructions"? The criteria need to be precise enough that when presented with a potential participant, everyone would agree about including or excluding the person. When you can count on understanding who is a participant, you can count on understanding the meaning and application of the findings to appropriate situations. When it is unclear who participated in the study, the applications of the findings also come into question.

PRACTICE REVIEWING METHODS AND RESULTS

Sometimes it is helpful to have models when learning a new skill. You are going to practice analyzing Methods and Results sections using an already-prepared summary so you can compare your analysis to an expert who conducted the same analysis.

Activity 3-5
Summarize Key Points

Worksheet: Examine the Similarities and Differences in the Summary Tables

The skill of summarizing the Methods and Results of a research article in a succinct table can be a great way to work in a study group with your colleagues because you can cover more material when everyone can see the overview quickly and don't have to page through the article as you go. It looks simple when you are reading a completed summary, but trying to figure out where to start on your own can be daunting.

Let's compare the two summary tables from Liu et al. (2013) and Berger et al. (2013). You will need to obtain the summary tables from the supplemental material about these articles on the following website: http://ajot.aotapress.net. Navigate to the article and then click on "Supplemental Materials."

Liu was interested in activities of daily living, while Berger was focused on leisure and socialization for adults with low vision, yet they have seven articles in common for their summary review. When we examine summary review tables like these, as readers we are grateful for the work to put all this reference material in one place for us.

These two tables, with some matching citations, give us a chance to see what details we really find useful since the authors presented the same material in two different ways. Being mindful of which details are helpful to you makes it easier to create summary tables for yourself.

Let's look at one reference to get started. Pankow, Luchins, Studebaker, and Chettleburgh (2004) is included in both tables. In Table 3-1 some of the comment boxes are completed for you. What would you say about the other components?

Now select two other pairs of articles that these reviews share and complete the worksheet with your study partners. Discuss your individual preferences and make notes about what you want to remember when you are making a summary review table.

Activity 3-6
Summarize Methods and Results

Worksheet: Summarize Intervention Studies

Review three articles from either Liu et al. (2013) or Berger et al. (2013) and complete the worksheet. As you read, mark the parts of the article that coincide with the headings on the worksheet, then complete the worksheet on the articles. In class with study partners and your teacher, compare what you wrote with what the authors wrote about these articles. What did you forget? Did you provide too many details?

Table 3-1

Examine the Similarities and Differences in the Summary Tables

Comparing the entries for: Pankow et al. (2004)

	From Liu et al. (2013)	From Berger et al. (2013)	My Comments
Level/design/ participants			
Study objectives	*Examine the effectiveness of a goal-attaining low vision rehabilitation program.*	*Determine whether a vision rehabilitation program would improve independent functioning in older adults with visual impairments.*	*The Berger statement provides me with more details about the study in one statement: I feel unclear what a "goal-attaining…" program is (Liu).*
Intervention and outcome measures			*I like having the "control" group and outcome measures on a separate line so I can see it quickly (Berger).*
Results			
Study limitations			*They reported different things and I wanted to know all of them.*

Adapted from Liu et al. (2013) and Berger et al. (2013).

Now that you have practiced, you likely have a preference for certain methods. There are other methods as well. The appendices in Law and MacDermid (2014) provide several methods for your consideration. Professionals will find different formats useful for summarizing a study.

PRACTICING SUMMARIZING FINDINGS FROM A STUDY

When you read a research article, you must understand the findings and the meaning of the findings for practice situations. When you are in a practice situation, colleagues, families, and other care providers expect that you are familiar with the current literature. They want to know what the articles mean for their situation. Therefore, you need to understand how to translate the findings into regular words that you can share with others. One way to begin is to think about what you would say to a particular person (e.g., "I just read an article about what we are discussing, and their findings suggest we consider XXX in our interventions").

Professionals want clear, easy-to-understand guidelines about what to do to improve their practices based on the most recent evidence. We will call these summaries "Take-Home Messages" to remind ourselves to use understandable language. You will need to consider Take-Home Messages for your colleagues (within your discipline and from other disciplines), family members, other care providers, and those receiving your care.

When considering what you are going to write, think about these questions:

- What would you say to colleagues about how they might need to change their practices to gain the optimal benefit?
- What would you say to your team regarding the articles' findings based on the articles you have read?
- How would you extrapolate information from these articles to develop hypotheses for other populations than the ones that were studied?

Activity 3-7
Create Take-Home Messages From Research Articles

Worksheet: Write Brief Take-Home Messages

Read the following article, which examines the effectiveness of two interventions.

Peiris, C. L., Shields, N., Brusco, N. K., Watts, J. J., & Taylor, N. F. (2013). *Additional Saturday rehabilitation improves functional independence and quality of life and reduces length of stay: A randomized controlled trial.* BMC Medicine, 11(1), 1-11. https://doi.org/10.1186/1741-7015-11-198

Review Sidebar 3-1, which summarizes the parts of the article. We are only considering the immediate effects of the intervention; in the study they also examined long-term effects. We also are only considering the primary outcomes to make this activity more concise. Compare this summary to your understanding of the article from your reading.

Now complete the worksheet to design Take-Home Messages using this article as your source of information. Pretend that this is the only article about amount of rehabilitation, and only consider the immediate benefits (at discharge only) and primary outcomes (the FIM, the EQ-5D, and length of stay) to make the task a little easier.

Sidebar 3-1
Summary of Peiris et al. (2013)

Article Example

Peiris, C. L., Shields, N., Brusco, N. K., Watts, J. J., & Taylor, N. F. (2013). Additional Saturday rehabilitation improves functional independence and quality of life and reduces length of stay: A randomized controlled trial. *BMC Medicine, 11*(1), 1-11. https://doi.org/10.1186/1741-7015-11-198

Many inpatients receive little or no rehabilitation on weekends. Our aim was to determine what effect providing additional Saturday rehabilitation during inpatient rehabilitation had on functional independence, quality of life, and length of stay compared to 5 days per week of rehabilitation.

Research Question

What is the effect of providing additional Saturday rehabilitation service in inpatient rehabilitation on discharge outcomes of functional independence, quality of life, and length of stay?

Participants

996 patients provided informed consent

Inclusion:	18 years and older
	Admitted to rehabilitation
	Can have other orthopedic, neurological, or other conditions
	Can speak another language (use interpreter)
	Can have reduced cognition (next of kin provides consent)
Exclusion:	Admitted for geriatric evaluation and management
	Enrolled in another intervention trial
Instrument:	Functional Independence Measure (FIM)
	EuroQoL questionnaire (EQ-5D)
	Length of stay (number of overnight stays in rehab)

Procedure

They tracked patients admitted to their rehabilitation facilities for 1 year.

Treatment Conditions

Group 1: Usual care group, Monday to Friday rehabilitation
Group 2: Intervention group, Monday to Saturday rehabilitation

Results

Intervention group had higher FIM scores at discharge.
Intervention group had higher EQ-5D utility index scores.
Intervention group had a 2-day shorter length of stay.
Intervention group received an average of 53 minutes more of rehabilitation.

Activity 3-8
Share With Study Partners

Share your Take-Home Messages with your study partners and see how each of yours compared. Do you agree with each other about the findings? Did you say something that no one else said?

Revise your Take-Home Messages based on feedback.

Activity 3-9
Recognize the Strengths and Limitations of Research Articles

Worksheet: Identify Answerable and Unanswerable Questions

All research articles make a contribution and have limitations. Perhaps a group of articles is only about one age group and diagnosis—then we are not sure whether we can apply their findings to other age groups and other diagnoses. There will always be practice questions that can and cannot be answered by the available research. Sometimes researchers conduct studies about what can be answered, but that does not mean that studies reflect the only important topics for practice. Perhaps there are no measures to find out the answer to an important practice question. It might be that a population is so heterogeneous that it is hard to detect changes or discover who would or would not profit from an intervention. In practice, there will always be answerable and unanswerable questions. Advances in measurement, technology, and knowledge make more questions answerable.

Considering the Peiris et al. (2013) article, complete the worksheet about the answerable and unanswerable questions for practice. Meet with your study partners and compare your lists. Discuss the items that were unique on people's lists and add ideas to your original list.

SUMMARY

Now that you have a beginning understanding of the parts of articles and what they provide, you are ready to look at topical articles to derive meaning from a group of studies.

PRACTICE WITH AN ENTIRE ARTICLE

Now that you have practiced with parts of articles, let's take one article and look at several parts at one time.

Finlayson, M., Preissner, K., Cho, C., & Plow, M. (2011). Randomization trial of a teleconference-delivered fatigue management program for people with multiple sclerosis. Multiple Sclerosis Journal, 17(9), 1130-1140. https://doi.org/10.1177/1352458511404272

Finlayson et al. (2011) completed a randomized trial of a teleconference-delivered fatigue management intervention with people with multiple sclerosis (MS). This is a good article for novices to evidence-based practice because the article is clearly written, contains several types of statistical analyses, includes graphing, and has some thought-provoking ideas to pose for the future. Additionally, it addresses an emergent type of intervention, so it provides a look at a topic that is of interest to many professionals working with people who have variable access to services. The article is an intervention study; for this exercise we will focus on the structure of the article itself, rather than on the intervention.

Activity 3-10
Summarize an Article

Worksheet: Summarize the Characteristics of a Research Article

Complete the worksheet to summarize the key points of the Finlayson et al. (2011) article.

You can get most of the information for the worksheet from the Abstract, but you will also need to search through the Methods section to get some of the needed details from the study.

Examining the Introduction

During the Introduction, the reader expects to get an overview of the work in the area of interest that builds a case for the study. Since there is limited space, authors have to be selective about how they build their case.

Activity 3-11
Identify Themes

Worksheet: Summarize Themes in the Introduction

You can begin to look at the Introduction by looking for the overall themes. This study has three paragraphs leading to the statement of hypotheses of this study. Read each paragraph and write the theme of that paragraph; sometimes this helps you to see the key points of their argument.

Activity 3-12
Discuss the Introduction

Now meet with your study partners and discuss the themes you see in the Introduction. What argument are the authors trying to make? Did they convince you that the study would be an important contribution?

Framework for the Study

Finlayson et al. (2011) state three hypotheses for their study:

1. Individuals who participate in the program will report significantly reduced fatigue impact, reduced fatigue severity, and improved HRQOL [health-related quality of life] immediately post-intervention compared with individuals allocated to the wait-list control group.

2. Participants will report significantly reduced fatigue impact, reduced fatigue severity, and improved HRQOL after the intervention compared with beforehand.

3. Any improvements in fatigue impact, fatigue severity, and HRQOL will be maintained 6 months after the intervention.

As the reader, you will want to watch for study design, methods, and results that align with these hypotheses. Alignment is the only way researchers can answer their questions and test their hypotheses with confidence.

Analyzing the Methods Section of an Article

Participants

The authors tell you how they found individuals to participate in their study in the first part of this section. Then they tell you the inclusion criteria for participants.

Activity 3-13
Summarize Inclusion Criteria

Worksheet: Summarize the Inclusion Criteria

Summarize these participant criteria in the worksheet.

Measures

The authors list the outcome measures used in the study and summarize the validity and reliability of the measures to familiarize the reader with their assessments.

Activity 3-14
Find More Information About the Measures

Look up further information on one of the assessments to find out more about the measure. Be sure to include information about the measure's validity and reliability. Kramer and Grampurohit (2020) provide a summary of many measures used in applied science research and may be a good reference for practice settings.

Procedures

This study's procedures are included in the "trial design," "randomization," and "statistical methods" sections under Methods.

Results

The authors provide a combination of text, tables, and figures to report their results. This is a great strategy because it accommodates all types of readers (i.e., those that understand the text explanation, those that enjoy examining the numbers they reported, and those that prefer graphs to show relationships).

Understanding the Relationship Among Graphs, Tables, and Text

In the Finlayson et al. (2011) study, Figure 4 provides the detailed averages across all the testing periods for the summary statistics in Tables 1 and 2. These authors were efficient in their use of space by providing different numbers in tables and figures. They also labeled everything so you can look at each component across the tables and figures.

You will see in their Figure 4 that they graphed only five of the SF-36 test scores. These subtests showed the most changes, so they wanted to highlight them in the figure. You can see in their Table 4 that the five subtests graphed in Figure 4 show the highest pre-post differences. Look in Columns 2 and 4 of Table 4. Highlight the five subtests pictured in Figure 4 to see this pattern. Additionally, their Table 4 contains the 95% confidence intervals (95% CI). This means that about 95% of participants' scores would fall in this range. The CI gives you an idea whether the participants were really different or more alike.

Activity 3-15
Find the Text to Match the Tables and Figures

Find the text that explains their Table 3 and match up the text with the results on Table 3. Meet with your study partners and discuss how the tables and figures enhance the reporting of results.

Decoding the Text Results

Let's use the paragraph that starts with "Findings for Hypothesis 1…" on p. 1135 to examine the details of statistical results. In this paragraph, the authors are reporting about a specific analysis they did to understand their findings for their first hypothesis. You will note that they only report what they did and their findings—it is not appropriate to add interpretations to the Results section. This gives the reader the chance to study the results and create some preliminary ideas before reading what the authors are thinking (their interpretive ideas will be in the Discussion section to follow).

In the first sentence, they say "Findings for Hypothesis 1…", so the reader has to go back to the Introduction to be reminded about this hypothesis. Go back to p. 1131 and jot down Hypothesis 1 so you can use it as you look at the table of results.

The effectiveness analysis (comparing those people who got the intervention right away with those on the waitlist) is in the first set of columns on their Table 3. Look at the first three rows of numbers under "effectiveness analysis." You will see that there is an asterisk after the fourth number, or the "p" level. To make it easier for the reader, researchers mark the scores that meet significant statistical difference standards. YEA!

You will see four sets of numbers across the columns. When you read the title of the table, it tells you these are "within person differences." This means that they subtracted each person's Week 1 (pre) from Week 7 (post) scores and analyzed this difference. Those numbers in the "mean" column tell you how much people changed, on average. Since these first sets of numbers are about fatigue, going down is a good outcome.

The second column tells us the standard deviation. We can see how spread apart the scores are from this number. Which FIS subscore has the largest variation? Discuss with your study partners why you think this score is so variable compared to the others.

The last two columns provide the statistics from the analysis. The "t" score is the actual calculation, and the p score tells us whether the t score is big enough to matter. You can see at the bottom of the table that the authors made adjustments from the traditional $p < .05$ criteria. Since they had many comparisons, they made it harder to meet the significance standard. This is a careful step that researchers use to make sure they aren't saying too many things changed, when some could have been by chance.

It is so interesting in this study that the **impact** of fatigue on people's lives seemed to change more than their actual fatigue severity (FSS). You will have to wait till the Discussion to find out what the authors think about this. All they say here is "similar findings were not observed for FSS …" That is because we only report the facts in Results. We will see what the authors have to say about this in the Discussion.

There are other results in this study. We just want you to have a beginning experience linking the text to the tables and figures here. We will have many more opportunities in future units. Your faculty may wish to delve deeper into these results in group discussion.

Since the reader won't find out what the authors think of this finding until the Discussion, the reader can reflect on what this finding might mean. This pattern of fatigue impact compared to fatigue severity is intriguing. Discuss with your study partners all the reasons you think this might have happened. (Aren't you excited to know what the authors think too?)

Activity 3-16
Discuss the Text of the Results

Meet with study partners to examine other paragraphs in the Results section. Discuss what the authors are telling the readers. Hypothesize what the results might mean so you can compare to the authors' ideas in the discussion.

Activity 3-17
Answer Research Questions

These authors set out three hypotheses for the study. Meet with your study partners to identify which paragraphs, tables, and graphs address each of the three hypotheses. Discuss whether you felt that the authors addressed each of the aims and what the answer to their hypotheses would be.

Discussion

In the Discussion section, the reader expects the authors to examine their findings and derive meaning from them. These authors provide a clear map for the reader about the progression of their Discussion. They use key phrases to alert the reader (e.g., "The findings of Hypothesis 1…" on p. 1138). These marker phrases help the reader to frame the Discussion. They do provide a clear statement about Hypothesis 2, but you will have to study a little more to find the discussion about Hypothesis 3. Remind yourself about Hypothesis 3, and then work with study partners to find the discussion points about this hypothesis.

Many times sections of the Discussion will coincide with particular results. We examined the Results paragraph about their Hypothesis 1, so let's look at the Discussion about this finding. The authors restate the finding in the first sentence, and then go on to tell the reader what they think this means. They say that perhaps their inclusion criteria made it harder to see a change in fatigue severity. They also talk about underlying pathology of the condition being harder to influence in the type of intervention they tested. The next paragraph about Hypothesis 1 outlines more factors. Meet with your study partners to discuss which ideas were on your lists when you had only the results to consider. We are betting you had some of the same ideas as the authors! Now that was worth waiting for, wasn't it?

Activity 3-18
Link Discussion With Results

Find other sections of the Discussion that you can link to sections of the Results. Discuss with your study partners to make sure you understand the authors' conclusions and hypotheses. Do you have alternate interpretations of the data? What other explanations could be posed? Are the authors revealing any biases in their Discussion?

Activity 3-19
Handle Anomalous Data

Worksheet: Reactions to New Data

The findings from this article may challenge some of your current beliefs. Refer to your Executive Summary (see Sidebar 2-1) of the Chinn and Brewer (1993) article to decide where your reactions to the article findings are occurring. Bring these issues up with your study partners.

Developing Take-Home Messages

The final step in the analysis process for evidence-based practice is to summarize the findings for those who need to use the ideas to improve their practices. Professionals want clear, easy-to-understand guidelines about what to do. We will call these summaries "Take-Home Messages" to remind ourselves to use understandable language. You will need to consider Take-Home Messages for your colleagues (within your discipline and from other disciplines), family members, other care providers, and those receiving your care. In the case of this article, think about how you would tell clients with MS how fatigue might affect them, and why you want to have some sessions to talk with them about strategies.

Activity 3-20
Develop Take-Home Messages

Worksheet: Create Take-Home Messages

Consider people with MS as the focus of your attention and create some Take-Home Messages for them. Pretend that the article you read was the **definitive** article on the topic.

When considering what you are going to write, think about these questions:

- What would you say to a client or family about how they might need to change their routines to gain the optimal benefit?
- What would you say to your team in a meeting about your client with MS regarding the article's findings (Finlayson et al., 2011)?
- How would you extrapolate information from this article to develop hypotheses for other populations than MS?

Summary

Sometimes taking the time to go through one article helps develop skills for deriving meaning for evidence-based practice. In this unit, you learned about the parts of research articles and what to expect from each part. Using this information, professionals can take advantage of what the literature has available to make their practices evidence based.

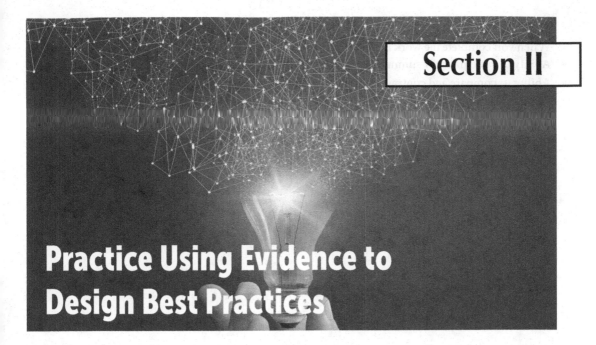

Practice Using Evidence to Design Best Practices

It is all well and good to learn research and evidence concepts, but this doesn't automatically enable professionals to use these concepts to affect their everyday practices. If you want to be an evidence-based practitioner, you must practice how to harness ideas from the literature. With the tools from Section I, we can begin looking at groups of articles about similar topics and make decisions about what their findings tell us about our professional practices.

In this section, you will examine several selections of articles on particular topics, and then develop "Take-Home Messages" from the articles. You will consider what you would say to various audiences about the topics, including colleagues on your team, family members, and other people or agencies you serve. In each unit, you will explore several topics that are applicable to a wide range of practice situations. Then, you will have some opportunities to apply the same strategies to some articles that will inform your areas of practice.

We cover a range of subjects in the units to expose you to various practice areas, age groups, and research methods and designs. There is no way to cover all possible areas of interest for students and faculty. You and your faculty members may have an interest in other topics; in this case, use the formats from these units to design your own personalized exploration of a topic.

FORMAT FOR WORK IN SECTION II

Throughout Section II, you will follow the same format for your work. You will read a few articles about a similar topic, complete a summary worksheet on those articles, identify similarities and differences among the articles, and get feedback from study partners. You will also examine research designs, statistical procedures, reporting of results, and interpreting discussions in the articles as well. You will have a nice collection of Take-Home Messages for your practice when you complete the work of Section II. You will also have an established pattern of systematic analysis you can use for future articles that become available, making your work more efficient.

When you complete the work in Section II, you will have the following skills and competencies:

- Ability to systematically summarize the Methods and Results of research articles
- Ability to compare and contrast findings across articles on similar topics
- Ability to derive meaning from Methods, Designs, Results, and Discussions in research articles
- Ability to discuss insights with colleagues to refine understanding about research findings
- Ability to construct Take-Home Messages for communities of interest

Please feel free to use the formats from these units to explore other topics of your interest.

Examining Evidence Related to Assistive Devices and Environmental Adaptations

During this unit, you will explore some evidence about the impact of technology on a person's ability to participate in their everyday life. This topic is applicable to a wide range of populations and settings, and so can be informative to many types of practice. Using technology to support everyday life provides people with direct access to the activities they want and need to do each day; understanding evidence about what, how, and when to apply various technologies can improve our effectiveness at supporting people within their lives.

Technology is becoming ubiquitous in our lives and in the lives of the people we serve. We make recommendations about using technologies of all kinds as adaptations, as intervention tools, and as mediums through which services can be delivered. Perhaps we need to wonder which technologies are most helpful, or which are most cumbersome even though they work when someone actually uses them. Perhaps some technologies simply don't work in the sense that they take too much time, are not accessible to everyone, or the technology replaces part of an activity that was satisfying for the person.

So, let's delve into this literature and find out what the researchers and their participants have to say about the use of technology to support people's lives.

When you complete the work for this unit, you will have the following skills and competencies:

- Understanding how literature may contribute to your effectiveness at supporting people to participate in their everyday lives
- Recognizing that diverse literature suggests enduring themes related to technology
- Articulating how to find other articles that would contribute to your knowledge about this topic
- Designing an optimal plan for your area of practice based on what you have read
- Constructing Take-Home Messages for various constituents so they understand quickly what the literature says about technology

You will be reviewing articles, creating summaries for comparison and contrast, gaining insights from your study partners, and creating Take-Home Messages for constituent groups.

Dunn, W., & Proffitt, R. *Bringing Evidence Into Everyday Practice: Practical Strategies for Health Care Professionals, Second Edition* (pp. 29-35).
© 2024 Taylor & Francis Group.

Activity 4-1
Read the Literature

Read the first five articles listed here. These articles will provide background for your work in this unit and will shed some light on the use of technology to support everyday life. For this unit, focus on the ways that technology contributes to participation and satisfaction in everyday life.

Bickmore, T. W., Caruso, L., Clough-Gorr, K., & Heeren, T. (2005). "It's just like you talk to a friend" relational agents for older adults. Interacting with Computers, 17, 711-735. https://doi.org/10.1016/j.intcom.2005.09.002

Campbell, R. J., & Nolfi, D. A. (2005). Teaching elderly adults to use the internet to access health care information: Before-after study. Journal of Medical Internet Research, 7(2), e19. https://doi.org/10.2196/jmir.7.2.e19

Demeris, G., Rantz, M. J., Aud, M. A., Marek, K. D., Tyrer, H. W., Skubic, M., & Hussam, A. A. (2004). Older adults' attitudes towards and perceptions of "smart home" technologies: A pilot study. Medical Informatics and the Internet in Medicine, 29(2), 87-94. https://doi.org/10.1080/14639230410001684387

Gellis, Z. D., Kenaley, B., McGinty, J., Bardelli, E., Davitt, J., & Ten Have, T. (2012). Outcomes of a telehealth intervention for homebound older adults with heart or chronic respiratory failure: A randomized controlled trial. The Gerontologist, 52(4), 541-552. https://doi.org/10.1093/geront/gnr134

Reeder, B., Demeris, G., & Marek, K. D. (2013). Older adults' satisfaction with a medication dispensing device in home care. Informatics for Health and Social Care, 38(3), 211-222. https://doi.org/10.3109/17538157.2012.741084

For later in the unit:

Yusif, S., Soar, J., & Hafeez-Baig, A. (2016). Older people, assistive technologies, and the barriers to adoption: A systematic review. International Journal of Medical Informatics, 94, 112-116. https://doi.org/10.1016/j.ijmedinf.2016.07.004

Activity 4-2
Examine Methods and Results Sections

Worksheet: Summarize the Characteristics of a Research Article

Create a summary table using the worksheet for these articles.

Summary tables show readers the most important aspects of studies. Locate a summary article in an area of your interest and see how they organize their tables. Make an organizational table that suits your learning and information needs.

LOOKING FOR PATTERNS AND THEMES

First, look for similarities and differences in the structures of the studies.

- Did they study the same populations?
- Did they use similar settings?
- Were the designs similar?
- How did the measures compare to each other?

The answers to these questions can help you understand differences in findings. For example, if one study says that a certain technology is effective and another study says no one uses that technology, you will need to examine these other factors to see what might have contributed to the differences. One study might have examined older adults living in a rural area with limited internet access, while another study might have examined a younger cohort. You can then hypothesize that devices are only effective with a certain group or when outcomes address only certain aspects of everyday life activities.

Now, think about the topic.

- What happened to your thinking from before and after reading the articles?
- How did your ideas change?
- Have you observed that professionals have incorporated these findings into their practices?
- Are you going to do anything differently now that you have read these studies?

Now, consider what questions are answerable or unanswerable from these studies.

Activity 4-3
Recognize Strengths and Limitations

Worksheet: Identify Answerable and Unanswerable Questions

All research articles make a contribution and have limitations. Perhaps a group of articles is only about one age group and diagnosis—then we are not sure whether we can apply their findings to other age groups and other diagnoses. There will always be practice questions that can and cannot be answered by the available research. Sometimes researchers conduct studies about what can be answered, but that does not mean that studies reflect the only important topics for practice. Perhaps there are no measures to find out the answer to an important practice question. It might be that a population is so heterogeneous that it is hard to detect changes or discover who would or would not profit from an intervention. In practice, there will always be answerable and unanswerable questions. Advances in measurement, technology, and knowledge make more questions answerable.

Considering this group of articles, complete the worksheet about the answerable and unanswerable questions for practice.

Activity 4-4
Discuss Ideas

Discuss your ideas and queries related to the questions above with your study partners.

Activity 4-5
Handle Anomalous Data

Worksheet: Reactions to New Data

The findings from these articles may challenge some of your current beliefs. Refer to your Executive Summary (see Sidebar 2-1) of the Chinn and Brewer (1993) article to decide where your reactions to the article findings are occurring. Bring these issues up with your study partners. Complete the worksheet with the technology findings on your mind. Be prepared to discuss the ideas you have with your study partners. Also consider what you might say to someone with each of the responses if you were in a conversation.

Activity 4-6
Expand the Evidence

Worksheet: Summarize the Characteristics of a Research Article

Obtain another article (i.e., in the past 5 years) that adds information to your understanding about this topic. Add this citation, etc., to your summary worksheet. Make copies of your article for your study partners.

Activity 4-7
Discuss Findings

Meet with your study partners and discuss your findings and reactions to the articles. Add your unique information to the discussion from the article you are contributing on the topic. Refine your notes based on your discussion.

These studies were a combination of experimental and descriptive designs, so we have a mix of information to deal with. The studies also included people with and without disabilities, which enable us to generalize the information across a wider group. In your practice, you might use the Demeris et al. (2004) findings to hypothesize that older adults want technology and devices that are intuitive to use and require minimal training. You could use the same framework and try to implement a new wearable technology in a nursing home setting. You could also add in information from the Gellis et al. (2012) study to see whether an intensive tutorial, training, and knowledge demonstration requirement leads to increased usability. These are examples of how to integrate the findings from these studies together and use them in new ways that inform your particular practice's issues. Be prepared to discuss other options with your study partners.

EXTENDING KNOWLEDGE ABOUT METHODS AND RESULTS

Every set of articles reflects an overall topic. Additionally, each article illustrates some unique features of studies and ways to report the methods and findings. By examining some aspects of each study, you will accumulate knowledge about designs and statistics while learning more about the evidence. This process will build your capacity as an evidence-based professional because when you encounter other articles with similar features, you will know how to incorporate the information in your decision making.

UNDERSTANDING HOW TO COMBINE EXPERIMENTAL AND DESCRIPTIVE DATA

You will notice that the first five articles about technology have a combination of experimental and descriptive studies. In this situation, you might be able to hypothesize about intervention options more directly by using the intervention studies as your basis for thinking. You can then use the descriptive study findings to expand your ideas about what conditions might need technology to increase life satisfaction for the people you serve. Perhaps a team will be able to identify criteria for recommending a device to an individual and criteria for **not** recommending a technology service or device.

Evidence Detective Tip

You can extend what you know from experimental studies by looking at the characteristics of descriptive studies on the same topic.

Think about how you would reorganize your thinking about recommending technologies. How will you individualize your choices about different technologies? How will your choices be different depending on how training is set up?

Activity 4-8
Combine Experimental and Descriptive Data

Worksheet: Examine Ways to Expand Knowledge About Assistive Devices

Some of the studies in this unit address issues related to assistive devices. Two of the studies are experimental (Campbell & Nolfi, 2005; Gellis et al., 2012). Let's look at the insights we have gained from these two intervention studies, and then consider how to expand our knowledge about technology using the other three descriptive studies you read.

In the first column of the worksheet, identify a finding from one of the intervention studies. Now review the three descriptive studies' findings to identify something from these studies that could expand your ideas from the experimental studies. You will use these ideas in your discussion group with your study partners. One example is completed on the worksheet to provide a model for your work.

In this example, we are expanding the idea of usability and follow-up using the additional information from the descriptive studies. When trying these ideas, a therapist would collect data with the people on the therapist's caseload to see if this new application of the knowledge is also effective.

Now complete a few more rows with your ideas and be prepared to discuss them with your study partners. There are several ways to organize the themes from these studies—there is not only one way that is correct.

Activity 4-9
Discuss Organizing Themes

When you meet with your study partners, share your different ways of organizing the themes and discuss how you identified these themes.

Activity 4-10
Develop Take-Home Messages
Worksheet: Create Take-Home Messages

The final step in the analysis process for evidence-based practice is to summarize the findings for those who need to use the ideas to improve their practices. Professionals want clear, easy-to-understand guidelines about what to do. We will call these summaries "Take-Home Messages" to remind ourselves to use understandable language. You will need to consider Take-Home Messages for your colleagues (within your discipline and from other disciplines), family members, other care providers, and those receiving your care.

Select a constituent group as the focus of your attention and create some Take-Home Messages for them. Pretend that the articles you read were the **definitive** articles on the topic. Use the worksheet to summarize your work.

When considering what you are going to write, think about these questions:
- What would you say to family members about how your choices are aligned with evidence to gain the optimal benefit for their loved one?
- What criteria would you use to decide whether the intervention is working with this person? (This helps you decide whether to continue or think of another approach.)
- What would you say to your team regarding the articles' findings based on the articles you have read?
- How would you extrapolate information from these articles to develop hypotheses for populations other than the ones that were studied?

Activity 4-11
Consider "Smart" Devices

Worksheet. Integrate Data About Smart Devices From a Systematic Review With an Intervention Study

We also included two articles about "smart" devices in this unit because this is an adaptation-specific category of technology to support people in their everyday lives. "Smart" technologies often are internet-enabled devices that can be controlled by the individual as well as through timers and schedules. One article is a systematic review (Yusif et al., 2016), and the other article is a descriptive study (Reeder et al., 2013).

Using the worksheet, map the findings from Reeder et al. (2013) against the three barriers from the list of barriers from the Yusif et al. (2016) article. Be prepared to discuss your insights with your study partners.

The Reeder et al. (2013) article was not included in the scoping review. Both articles are about older adults' attitudes toward devices, so why was the Reeder et al. (2013) paper excluded? The way you find out about this is by looking at the criteria Yusif et al. (2016) used to select their articles. In Section 2.2.2 under "Exclusion Criteria," the authors state that they excluded studies about "Health Information Technology"-related studies. What characteristics of the medication-dispensing device meet these criteria? Do you think they should have included or excluded the Reeder et al. (2013) article?

Finally, consider what the Reeder et al. (2013) study adds to the story from the systematic review article. Discuss your ideas with your study partners.

SUMMARY

In this unit, you reviewed literature related to use of technology by older adults. This information enables professionals to make informed choices about how to select, train, and recommend these technologies to support a satisfying life.

Examining Evidence Related to the Use of Compensatory Strategies

During this unit, you will explore some evidence about the use of compensatory strategies to support participation. Many times, professionals focus their attention on changing the person's skills and abilities so the person can participate more effectively. Another option in intervention is to adjust environments and activities so that they are more "friendly" to the person; this supports successful participation as well.

We have two articles in this unit that inform our decisions about changing specific situations to support people's participation. Both articles studied application of compensatory strategies with people who have schizophrenia, but we could also study this topic with other populations and other age groups.

When you complete the work for this unit, you will have the following skills and competencies:
- Understanding how this literature may contribute to our knowledge about effectiveness
- Articulating how to find other articles that would contribute to your knowledge about this topic
- Designing an evidence-based plan for your area of practice based on what you have read
- Constructing Take-Home Messages for various constituents so they understand quickly what the literature says about the topic

You will be reviewing articles, creating summaries for comparison and contrast, gaining insights from your study partners, and creating Take-Home Messages for constituent groups.

Activity 5-1
Read the Literature

Read the articles listed here. These articles shed some light on use of compensatory strategies to support participation. For this exercise, focus on how they provided the supports and what measures they used to determine effectiveness.

Dunn, W., & Proffitt, R. *Bringing Evidence Into Everyday Practice: Practical Strategies for Health Care Professionals, Second Edition* (pp. 37-41).

Mendella, P. D., Burton, C. Z., Tasca, G. A., Roy, P., St. Louis, L., & Twamley, E. W. (2015). *Compensatory cognitive training for people with first-episode schizophrenia: Results from a pilot randomized controlled trial.* Schizophrenia Research, 162(1-3), 108-111. https://doi. org/10.1016/j.schres.2015.01.016

Velligan, D. I., Mueller, J., Wang, M., Dicocco, M., Diamond, P. M., Maples, N. J., & Davis, B. (2006). *Use of environmental supports among patients with schizophrenia.* Psychiatric Services, 57(2), 219-224. https://doi.org/10.1176/appi.ps.57.2.219

Activity 5-2
Summarize Methods and Results

Worksheet: Summarize the Characteristics of a Research Article

Create a summary table using the worksheet for these articles. Now find two more articles that provide additional information about compensatory methods for people with schizophrenia and include them on the worksheet.

Summary tables show readers the most important aspects of studies. You can find tables like the one on the worksheet in any article that is summarizing the literature in an area. You might find a different style that fits your learning and information needs in the literature.

LOOKING FOR PATTERNS AND THEMES

First, look for similarities and differences in the structures of the studies.

- Did they study the same populations?
- Did they use similar settings?
- Were the designs similar?
- How did the measures compare to each other?

The answer to these questions can help you understand differences in findings. For example, one study examined three conditions and the more recent study used two conditions; you will need to consider why this change occurred. Did the earlier study inform this decision? In these studies, there are some similar and some unique measures. How do the measures lead to similar or different results?

Now, think about the topic.

- What happened to your thinking from before and after reading the articles?
- How did your ideas change?
- Have you observed that professionals have incorporated these findings into their practices?
- Are you going to do anything differently now that you have read these studies?

These questions enable you to examine how the findings affected yours and others' thinking about practice. A great study that professionals are skeptical about will not have an impact on the practices. As professionals, we need to understand the reasons why people may or may not adopt a strategy that has been shown effective through a research study.

Now, consider what questions are answerable or unanswerable from these studies.

Activity 5-3
Recognize Strengths and Limitations

Worksheet: Identify Answerable and Unanswerable Questions

All research articles make a contribution and have limitations. Perhaps a group of articles is only about one age group and diagnosis—then we are not sure whether we can apply their findings to other age groups and other diagnoses. There will always be practice questions that can and cannot be answered by the available research. Sometimes researchers conduct studies about what can be answered, but that does not mean that studies reflect the only important topics for practice. Perhaps there are no measures to find out the answer to an important practice question. It might be that a population is so heterogeneous that it is hard to detect changes or discover who would or would not profit from an intervention. In practice, there will always be answerable and unanswerable questions. Advances in measurement, technology, and knowledge make more questions answerable.

Considering this group of articles, complete the worksheet about the answerable and unanswerable questions for practice.

Evidence Detective Tip
You can combine findings from different topics and populations
to gain a broader view.

Activity 5-4
Handle Anomalous Data

Worksheet: Reactions to New Data

The findings from these articles may challenge some of your current beliefs. Refer to your Executive Summary (see Sidebar 2-1) of the Chinn and Brewer (1993) article to decide where your reactions to the article findings are occurring. Bring these issues up with your study partners.

Activity 5-5
Discuss Ideas

Meet with your study partners and discuss the findings and your reactions to the articles. Add your unique information to the discussion from the articles you are contributing on the topic. Refine your notes based on your discussion.

Here are some questions to get you started:
- Why do you think that the more recent study only used two conditions?
- How did two or three conditions affect the findings?

- Why do you think that the group receiving generic adaptations in the Velligan et al. (2006) study had such a different outcome compared to the others?
- How could you apply these findings to other populations?

LINKING EVIDENCE FROM DIFFERENT WORLDS

Sometimes you can find helpful information about a problem in practice in a place you wouldn't expect. For example, in this unit you are working on studies that show creating specifically tailored cognitive adaptations increase a person with schizophrenia's ability to participate. In a previous unit, you examined studies that tested the impact of assistive devices: some participants had physical impairments, others were older adults who needed some adaptations. If you are in a practice that serves people with severe mental illness, you may not think to look at the older adult or physical disability literature, and yet, there may be some helpful information in all these places for several areas of practice.

Activity 5-6
Link Evidence Across Populations

Worksheet: Look for Themes Across Studies: Part 1

Worksheet: Look for Themes Across Studies: Part 2

Working with your study partners, identify themes from the combined list of articles in this unit and the articles from Unit 4. What are some common themes across all studies? What is a finding from one group that could inform (and hopefully improve) the interventions for another group? For example, are there some findings from the cognitive adaptations studies that could improve technology training for older adults? Complete the two worksheets on your own, and then meet with your study partners to discuss what each of you thought about. Take notes to refine your own thinking. Both worksheets have been started for you.

Activity 5-7
Develop Take-Home Messages

Worksheet: Create Take-Home Messages

The final step in the analysis process for evidence-based practice is to summarize the findings for those who need to use the ideas to improve their practices. Professionals want clear, easy-to-understand guidelines about what to do. We will call these summaries "Take-Home Messages" to remind ourselves to use understandable language. You will need to consider Take-Home Messages for your colleagues (within your discipline and from other disciplines), family members, other care providers, and those receiving your care.

Select two constituent groups as the focus of your attention and create some Take-Home Messages for them. Pretend that the articles you read were the **definitive** articles on the topic. Use the worksheet to summarize your work.

When considering what you are going to write, think about these questions:

- What would you say to colleagues about how they might need to change their practices to gain the optimal benefit?
- What would you say to your team regarding the articles' findings based on the articles you have read?
- How would you extrapolate information from these articles to develop hypotheses for populations other than the ones that were studied?

SUMMARY

During this unit, you learned about the use of compensatory strategies to support participation. This evidence revealed the impact that changing environments and activities can have on participation. You also practiced integrating articles from this unit with the assistive device articles to gain a broader evidence-based perspective.

Examining Evidence Related to Caregiving

During this unit, you will explore some evidence about how caregiving affects people. This topic is interesting because we can study it across age groups and diagnoses. Many situations require someone to be a caregiver; for example, adults care for their own children, their partners, and their parents. In your practice you are likely to encounter people who are providing everyday care for someone you are serving in your professional role. Even though many systems require us to focus on a specific person who has an injury, disease, or disability, to provide best practice care we must also understand how to support and guide the friends and family who are or will be responsible for the target person in their everyday lives.

So, what does the literature tell us about the experience of caregiving? With these insights, what will we need to change about our approach to those providing care as a means for supporting the person we are serving?

We hope you are also curious about what you will find. Perhaps you are wondering whether people caring for adults have the same issues as people caring for children. Perhaps you want to know about caregiving that spans a short or long period of time. Jot down your ideas before you read, this will enable you to reflect on the literature in a more specific way.

When you complete the work for this unit, you will have the following skills and competencies:

- Understanding how caregiver literature may contribute to your effectiveness for serving the person and their friends and family
- Recognizing themes in diverse literature that suggest enduring themes related to caregiving
- Articulating how to find other articles that would contribute to your knowledge about this topic
- Designing an optimal plan for your area of practice based on what you have read
- Constructing Take-Home Messages for various constituents so they understand quickly what the literature says about caregiving

You will be reviewing articles, creating summaries for comparison and contrast, gaining insights from your study partners, and creating Take-Home Messages for constituent groups.

Dunn, W., & Proffitt, R. *Bringing Evidence Into Everyday Practice: Practical Strategies for Health Care Professionals, Second Edition* (pp. 43-48).
© 2024 Taylor & Francis Group.

Activity 6-1
Read the Literature

Read the articles listed here. These articles shed some light on the experience of caregiving. For this unit, focus on the issues of barriers and solutions that caregivers report about their experiences.

Huang, C., Yen, H., Tseng, M., Tung, L., Chen, Y., & Chen, K. (2014). *Impacts of autistic behaviors, emotional and behavioral problems on parenting stress in caregivers of children with autism.* Journal of Autism and Developmental Disorders, 44(6), 1383-1390. https://doi.org/10.1007/s10803-013-2000-y

Kim, H., Chang, M., Rose, K., & Kim, S. (2012). *Predictors of caregiver burden in caregivers of individuals with dementia.* Journal of Advanced Nursing, 68(4), 846-855. https://doi.org/10.1111/j.1365-2648.2011.05787.x

Northouse, L. L., Katapodi, M. C., Schafenacker, A. M., & Weiss, D. (2012). *The impact of caregiving on the psychological well-being of family caregivers and cancer patients.* Seminars in Oncology Nursing, 28(4), 236-245. https://doi.org/10.1016/j.soncn.2012.09.006

Activity 6-2
Summarize Methods and Results

Worksheet: Summarize the Characteristics of a Research Article

Create a summary table using the worksheet for these articles.

Summary tables show readers the most important aspects of studies. By taking the most important information from each article, it is easier to see across studies and look for patterns and themes.

LOOKING FOR PATTERNS AND THEMES

First, look for similarities and differences in the structures of the studies.
- Did they study the same populations?
- Did they use similar settings?
- Were the designs similar?
- How did the measures compare to each other?

The answer to these questions can help you understand differences in findings. For example, if one study says an intervention worked and another study says it did not, you will need to examine these other factors to see what might have contributed to the differences. One study might have examined caregiving of children and another the caregiving of adults. You can then hypothesize that the intervention is only effective with a certain group or when outcomes are measured in a certain way.

Now, think about the topic.

- What happened to your thinking from before and after reading the articles?
- How did your ideas change?
- Have you observed that professionals have incorporated these findings into their practices?
- Are you going to do anything differently now that you have read these studies?

Now, consider what questions are answerable or unanswerable from these studies.

Activity 6-3
Recognize Strengths and Limitations

Worksheet: Identify Answerable and Unanswerable Questions

All research articles make a contribution and have limitations. Perhaps a group of articles is only about one age group and diagnosis—then we are not sure whether we can apply their findings to other age groups and other diagnoses. There will always be practice questions that can and cannot be answered by the available research. Sometimes researchers conduct studies about what can be answered, but that does not mean that studies reflect the only important topics for practice. Perhaps there are no measures to find out the answer to an important practice question. It might be that a population is so heterogeneous that it is hard to detect changes or discover who would or would not profit from an intervention. In practice, there will always be answerable and unanswerable questions. Advances in measurement, technology, and knowledge make more questions answerable.

Considering this group of articles, complete the worksheet about the answerable and unanswerable questions for practice.

Activity 6-4
Handle Anomalous Data

Worksheet: Reactions to New Data

The findings from these articles may challenge some of your current beliefs. Refer to your Executive Summary (see Sidebar 2-1) of the Chinn and Brewer (1993) article to decide where your reactions to the article findings are occurring. Bring these issues up with your study partners.

Activity 6-5
Expand the Evidence

Worksheet: Summarize the Characteristics of a Research Article

Obtain another article (i.e., in the past 5 years) that adds information to your understanding about this topic. Add this citation, etc., to your summary worksheet. Make copies of your article for your study partners.

Activity 6-6
Discuss Ideas

Meet with your study partners and discuss your findings and reactions to the articles. Add your unique information to the discussion from the article you are contributing on the topic. Refine your notes based on your discussion.

Some of the studies were about caring for adults and the others were about caring for children; your additional studies likely covered the life span as well. The three original studies also covered many disabilities, and yet we could identify common themes within the caregiving experience. Discuss your thoughts and insights with your study partners.

EXTENDING KNOWLEDGE ABOUT
METHODS AND RESULTS

Every set of articles reflects an overall topic. Additionally, each article illustrates some unique features of studies and ways to report the methods and findings. By examining some aspects of each study, you will accumulate knowledge about designs and statistics while learning more about the evidence. This process will build your capacity as an evidence-based professional because when you encounter other articles with similar features, you will know how to use the information in your decision making.

Evidence Detective Tip

Descriptive studies provide insights to an experience, condition, or situation
that can refine your practices.

UNDERSTANDING HOW TO USE
EVIDENCE FROM VARIED STUDIES

Each of these studies reported themes they derived from their interviews and data collection. Let's take a little time to look at the themes in more detail.

Activity 6-7
Identify Themes

Worksheet. Find Similarities in Conceptual Themes
Worksheet: Find Unique Themes Across Studies

Make a list of the themes reported from each study using the worksheets. When you see something reported in more than one study, write down the concept or idea in the first column of the Similarities worksheet. Jot down what each author had to say about that concept. Go back to the first column and write a short rationale for clustering these themes together. Keep doing this until you don't see any more concepts that they share. Then look at unique concepts from each article using the Find Unique Themes Across Studies worksheet—do you think these unique features are related to the way the researchers conducted their study, are they about the population, or something else?

This process helps you to see what may be universal about the caregiver experience and what might be unique to certain situations. In the themes you created on the Find Similarities in Conceptual Themes worksheet, perhaps you saw that all three studies contain some discussion about caregivers' feelings about their role. Quotations from caregivers could also be added for validation.

There are several ways to organize the themes from these studies; there is not only one way that is correct. When you meet with your study partners, share your different ways of organizing the themes and discuss how you identified these themes.

Activity 6-8
Address Themes

Think about how you might address some of the common themes in your practice. For example, since we saw a theme of "interaction between how the person is doing and how the caregiver feels," what might you put into place ahead of time to ensure that caregivers are prepared for this feeling? Be prepared to discuss your strategies with your study partners.

Activity 6-9
Develop Take-Home Messages

Worksheet: Create Take-Home Messages

The final step in the analysis process for evidence-based practice is to summarize the findings for those who need to use the ideas to improve their practices. Professionals want clear, easy-to-understand guidelines about what to do. We will call these summaries "Take-Home Messages" to remind ourselves to use understandable language. You will need to consider Take-Home Messages for your colleagues (within your discipline and from other disciplines), family members, other care providers, and those receiving your care.

Select two constituent groups as the focus of your attention and create some Take-Home Messages for them. Pretend that the articles you read were the **definitive** articles on the topic. Use the worksheet to summarize your work.

When considering what you are going to write, think about these questions:

- What would you say to colleagues about how they might need to change their practices to gain the optimal benefit?
- What would you say to your team regarding the articles' findings based on the articles you have read?
- How would you extrapolate information from these articles to develop hypotheses for other populations than the ones that were studied?

Summary

In this unit, you learned about the experience of caregiving. The articles were descriptive in nature, and so provided a picture of caregiving from various points of view. These perspectives are useful to professionals in practice because they remind us about all the people we serve.

Examining Evidence Related to Sensory Processing Patterns

During this unit, you will explore some evidence about the various ways that people are exploring sensory processing patterns as an important factor in understanding behavior. There is a growing body of evidence using advanced statistical methods to identify the variability within groups of people that we used to see as homogeneous. For example, research into the characteristics of autism frequently uses the diagnosis of autism as an inclusion criterion without consideration to the fact that even within the group called "autistic," there are lots of individual differences. When we know more about individual differences, we can create more precise intervention strategies, and have a better chance at supporting that person, the family, and their care team.

The articles you will review in this unit have some features that are quite advanced for novice learners. We will focus our attention on specific aspects of these articles, trusting that the researchers did the studies properly and are reporting the best results possible. If this is an area of interest for you, talk with your faculty about how to learn more about the approaches in these studies.

When you complete the work for this unit, you will have the following skills and competencies:
- Understanding how this literature might support development of individualized interventions
- Hypothesizing how studies of different age groups might weave a cohesive story together
- Linking outcome statements with the literature and rationale supporting this outcome
- Constructing Take-Home Messages for families about what to expect as their children grow

You will be reviewing articles, creating summaries for comparison and contrast, writing rationales for conclusions that researchers have made, gaining insights from your study partners, and creating Take-Home Messages for constituent groups.

Dunn, W., & Proffitt, R. *Bringing Evidence Into Everyday Practice: Practical Strategies for Health Care Professionals, Second Edition* (pp. 49-55).

Activity 7-1
Read the Literature

Read the abstracts, identify the research questions or hypotheses, and skim the designated sections of the articles listed below.

DeSantis, A., Harkins, D., Tronick, E., Kaplan, E., & Beeghly, M. (2011). *Exploring an integrative model of infant behavior: What is the relationship among temperament, sensory processing, and neurobehavioral measures?* Infant Behavior and Development, 34(2), 280-292. https://doi.org/10.1016/j.infbeh.2011.01.003

- Participants: Section 2.1
- Table 2: Subscales Explained
- "An Integrated Model of Infant Behavior" (under Results)
- Discussion 4
- Tables 4 and 5

Lane, A. E., Molloy, C. A., & Bishop, S. L. (2014). *Classification of children with autism spectrum disorder by sensory subtype: A case for sensory-based phenotypes.* Autism Research, 7(3), 322-333. https://doi.org/10.1002/aur.1368

- Participants (under Methods)
- Sensory subtypes (under Results)
- Discussion

Little, L. M., Dean, E., Tomchek, S. D., & Dunn, W. (2016). *Classifying sensory profiles of children in the general population.* Child: Care, Health and Development, 43(1), 81-88. https://doi.org/10.1111/cch.12391

- Participants (under Methods)
- Figure 1 and the text explanation of this figure
- Results
- Discussion
- Key Messages

Tomchek, S., Little, L. M., Myers, J., & Dunn, W. (2018). *Sensory subtypes in preschool aged children with autism spectrum disorder.* Journal of Autism and Developmental Disorders, 48(6), 2139-2147. https://doi.org/10.1007/s10803-018-3468-2

- Participants (under Methods)
- Figures 1 and 2 and the text explanation of these figures
- Results (starting on p. 2143)
- Discussion

Uljarevic, M., Lane, A., Kelly, A., & Leekam, S. (2016). *Sensory subtypes and anxiety in older children and adolescents with autism spectrum disorder.* Autism Research, 9(10), 1073-1078. https://doi.org/10.1002/aur.1602

- Participants (under Methods)
- Results: Aim 1: Sensory Subtypes
- Discussion

These articles describe distinct profiles for infants, children, and adolescents related to sensory processing. Don't get bogged down in technical details; rather, look at the overall factors and profiles described in each article.

Activity 7-2
Summarize Factors and Profiles
Worksheet: Summarize the Characteristics of a Research Article

Create a summary table using the worksheet for these articles.

Tables with key points allow us to see the most important aspects of studies.

For these studies, we are interested in how the factors and profiles compare and contrast to each other.

LOOKING FOR PATTERNS AND THEMES

First, look for similarities and differences in the studies.

- How do the populations compare? How might this make a difference?
- How do the research questions align or diverge?
- What is similar or distinct about the different factors and profiles?

The answers to these questions can help you understand how to use the findings. For example, these studies used different age groups. What does this mean as you think about what sensory behaviors to look for when observing a child? How do these studies enable generalization? What do the studies have in common? You can use the patterns you see to begin formulating hypotheses for your practice.

Now, think about the topic.

- What happened to your thinking from before and after reading the articles?
- How did your ideas change?
- What might you do differently now that you have studied these articles?

Be prepared to discuss your ideas and queries with your study partners.

Now, consider what questions are answerable or unanswerable from these studies.

Activity 7-3
Recognize Strengths and Limitations
Worksheet: Identify Answerable and Unanswerable Questions

All research articles make a contribution and have limitations. Perhaps a group of articles is only about one age group and diagnosis—then we are not sure whether we can apply their findings to other age groups and other diagnoses. There will always be practice questions that can and cannot be answered by the available research. Sometimes researchers conduct studies about what can be answered, but that does not mean that studies reflect the only important topics for practice. Perhaps there are no measures to find out the answer to an important practice question. It might be that a population is so heterogeneous that it is hard to detect changes or discover who would or would not profit from an intervention. In practice, there will always be answerable and unanswerable questions. Advances in measurement, technology, and knowledge make more questions answerable.

Considering this group of articles, complete the worksheet about the answerable and unanswerable questions for practice.

Activity 7-4
Handle Anomalous Data

Worksheet: Reactions to New Data

The findings from these articles may challenge some of your current beliefs. Refer to your Executive Summary (see Sidebar 2-1) of the Chinn and Brewer (1993) article to decide where your reactions to the article findings are occurring. Bring these issues up with your study partners.

Be prepared to discuss the ideas you have with your study partners. Consider what you might say to someone with each of the responses if you were in a conversation.

Activity 7-5
Discuss Material

Meet with your study partners and discuss your insights and reactions to the articles. Refine your notes based on your discussion.

EXTEND KNOWLEDGE ABOUT
METHODS AND RESULTS

Every set of articles reflects an overall topic. In this set of articles, we see a similar approach with different populations, some different measures, and different age groups. We are going to look for threads that weave through the findings of these articles so you can develop a larger structure for using a set of articles.

These articles show how we can ask a similar question and, by looking at different samples of people and using different additional assessments, we can expand what we understand about development and adaptability. In this set of articles, sensory processing is at the center of everyone's exploration.

Evidence Detective Tip

There are families of statistical techniques that help us understand
how similar or distinct a set of characteristics are.

Activity 7-6
Practice With Your Study Partners

Work with your study partners to examine the tables, figures, and explanations of the profiles and factors.

- Which tables or figures were helpful to you? What made them helpful?
- Discuss which graphing strategy you like the most or least. Which article provided the clearest link between the numeric data and the illustrations? What was unclear? What suggestions would you make to improve one or all of these articles?
- Which descriptions of factors and profiles were most helpful to you? What made these descriptions more accessible to you? Did you notice too much jargon? Too little explanation?
- Remember your answers as you plan papers you have to write!

Activity 7-7
Practice With Your Study Partners

Worksheet: Create a Rationale for Summary Points From an Article

Look at the "Key Messages" box at the end of the Little et al. (2016) study.
Use the worksheet to do two things:

1. Restate the key point in everyday words for a neighbor or your grandparent.
2. Write a rationale (with references) for each key point they present. Discuss these with your study partners and/or present them in class.

Activity 7-8
Compare Features of Factors and Profiles

Worksheet: Summary Table for Sensory Processing Patterns

Meet with your study partners to compare and contrast the features of the profiles and factors. Use your summary table for sensory patterns articles to guide your thinking and discussion.

- How are the factors and profiles alike?
- How are the factors and profiles different?
- What is one distinct thing that each article contributes to our understanding about sensory processing patterns?

Activity 7-9
Trace the Factors and Profiles From Infancy to Adolescence

Meet with your study partners. Think about what profiles and factors are more alike. Start with DeSantis et al. (2011) who describe the infant factors. Select one of the factors as representative of a particular group of children. Now proceed through the articles related to age, and ask "What profile would these infants have when they are toddlers, preschoolers, children, or adolescents?"

DeSantis et al. (2011): Infants

Lane et al. (2014): Toddlers to school age

Little et al. (2016): Preschoolers to school age

Tomchek et al. (2018): Preschoolers

Uljarevic et al. (2016): Adolescents

With your study partners, write a paragraph describing this person you have tracked across development.

Activity 7-10
Know What the Public Might Know

The topic of sensory processing patterns has gotten a lot of public attention, so you will be able to find newspaper and magazine articles that discuss sensitivity particularly (e.g., Rix, 2007; Wallis, 2007). Find an article that journalistically reports about sensory experiences and share it with your study partners. Consider the following issues in your discussion.

- What are the differences between what actual professional authors say about their findings and what journalists say about the findings?
- In what ways might the public be served by this journalist report?
- In what ways might the public be misled by this journalist report?
- How do science and evidence advance with public articles such as this one?

Activity 7-11
Develop Take-Home Messages

Worksheet: Create Take-Home Messages

The final step in the analysis process for evidence-based practice is to summarize the findings for those who need to use the ideas to improve their practices. Professionals want clear, easy-to-understand guidelines about what to do. We will call these summaries "Take-Home Messages" to remind ourselves to use understandable language. You will need to consider Take-Home Messages for your colleagues (within your discipline and from other disciplines), family members, other care providers, and those receiving your care.

Select one constituent group as the focus of your attention and create some Take-Home Messages for them. Pretend that the articles you read were the **definitive** articles on the topic. Use the worksheet to summarize your work.

When considering what you are going to write, think about these questions:

- What would you say to colleagues about how they might need to change their practices to gain the optimal benefit?
- What would you say to your team regarding the articles' findings based on the articles you have read?
- How would you extrapolate information from these articles to develop hypotheses for populations other than the ones that were studied?

SUMMARY

In this unit, you learned about how sensory processing helps us understand individual differences. These individual differences are noticeable for infants, children, and adolescents and hold promise for planning the best interventions possible. We can also use this information to support families and educators as they care for children during active growth periods. Our contribution with these teams is to observe and interpret sensory behaviors to support a high quality of life and satisfying participation.

Examining Evidence Related to Constraint-Induced Therapy Interventions

During this unit, you will explore some evidence about the various ways that people are implementing constraint-induced therapy interventions. There is a growing body of evidence about constraint-induced therapy, so it is important for professionals providing service in rehabilitation to know what these researchers are finding and recommending for practice.

The articles you will review in this unit have some other features that will expand your understanding about how to read research papers, We will practice analyzing these features to give you some experience with the internal structure of research articles.

When you complete the work for this unit, you will have the following skills and competencies:

- Understanding how this literature may contribute to our knowledge about effective interventions
- Articulating how to find other articles that would contribute to your knowledge about the subject
- Identifying the parameters that seem to make the intervention effective and/or ineffective based on the evidence you have read
- Designing an optimal plan for your area of practice based on what you have read
- Constructing Take-Home Messages for various constituents so they understand quickly what the literature says about the subject

You will be reviewing articles, creating summaries for comparison and contrast, gaining insights from your study partners, and creating Take-Home Messages for constituent groups.

Dunn, W., & Proffitt, R. *Bringing Evidence Into Everyday Practice: Practical Strategies for Health Care Professionals, Second Edition* (pp. 57-63).

Activity 8-1
Read the Literature

Read the articles listed here.

Kitago, T., Liang, J., Huang, V. S., Hayes, S., Simon, P., Tenteromano, L., Lazar, R. M., Marshall, R. S., Mazzoni P., Lennihan, L., & Krakauer, J. W. (2013). Improvement after constraint-induced movement therapy: Recovery of normal motor control or task specific compensation? Neurorehabilitation and Neural Repair, 27(2), 99-109. https://doi.org/10.1177/1545968312452631

Klingels, K., Feys, H., Molenaers, G., Verbeke, G., Van Daele, S., Hoskens, J., Desloovere, K., & De Cock, P. (2013). Randomized trial of modified constraint-induced movement therapy with and without an intensive therapy program in children with unilateral cerebral palsy. Neurorehabilitation and Neural Repair, 27(9), 799-807. https://doi.org/10.1177/1545968313496322

The articles are from interdisciplinary literature and provide insights for professionals in several disciplines. Don't get bogged down in technical details; rather, look at the overall procedures and outcomes. When reading interdisciplinary literature in refereed journals, there must be some level of confidence that the blind review process led to the presentation of reasonable procedures to test the hypotheses.

Activity 8-2
Summarize Methods and Results

Worksheet: Summarize the Characteristics of a Research Article

Create a summary table using the worksheet for these articles.

Summary tables show readers the most important aspects of studies. Locate a summary article in an area of your interest and see how its tables are organized. Make an organizational table that suits your learning and information needs.

LOOKING FOR PATTERNS AND THEMES

First, look for similarities and differences in the structures of the studies.
- Did they study the same populations?
- Did they use similar settings?
- Were the designs similar?
- How did the measures compare to each other?

The answers to these questions can help you understand differences in findings. For example, these studies used different amounts of time and different methods for restraining movements. What does this mean as you think about evidence-based use of constraint-induced movement? One of the studies involved children; how does this enable generalization? What do the studies have in common? You can use the patterns you see to begin formulating hypotheses for your practice.

Now, think about the topic.
- What happened to your thinking from before and after reading the articles?
- How did your ideas change?

- Have you observed that professionals have incorporated these findings into their practices?
- Are you going to do anything differently now that you have read these studies?
  Be prepared to discuss your ideas and queries with your study partners.
  Now, consider what questions are answerable or unanswerable from these studies.

Activity 8-3
Recognize Strengths and Limitations

Worksheet: Identify Answerable and Unanswerable Questions

All research articles make a contribution and have limitations. Perhaps a group of articles is only about one age group and diagnosis—then we are not sure whether we can apply their findings to other age groups and other diagnoses. There will always be practice questions that can and cannot be answered by the available research. Sometimes researchers conduct studies about what can be answered, but that does not mean that studies reflect the only important topics for practice. Perhaps there are no measures to find out the answer to an important practice question. It might be that a population is so heterogeneous that it is hard to detect changes or discover who would or would not profit from an intervention. In practice, there will always be answerable and unanswerable questions. Advances in measurement, technology, and knowledge make more questions answerable.

Considering this group of articles, complete the worksheet about the answerable and unanswerable questions for practice.

Activity 8-4
Handle Anomalous Data

Worksheet: Reactions to New Data

The findings from these articles may challenge some of your current beliefs. Refer to your Executive Summary (see Sidebar 2-1) of the Chinn and Brewer (1993) article to decide where your reactions to the article findings are occurring. Bring these issues up with your study partners.

Be prepared to discuss the ideas you have with your study partners. Consider what you might say to someone with each of the responses if you were in a conversation.

Activity 8-5
Expand the Evidence

Worksheet: Summarize the Characteristics of a Research Article

Obtain another article (i.e., in the past 5 years) that adds information to your understanding about this topic. Add this citation, etc., to your summary worksheet. Make copies of your article for your study partners.

Activity 8-6
Discuss Material

Meet with your study partners and discuss your findings and reactions to the articles. Add your unique information to the discussion from the article you are contributing on the topic. Refine your notes based on your discussion.

EXTEND KNOWLEDGE ABOUT METHODS AND RESULTS

Every set of articles reflects an overall topic. Additionally, each article illustrates some unique features of studies and ways to report the methods and findings. By examining some aspects of each study, you will accumulate knowledge about designs and statistics while learning more about the evidence. This process will build your capacity as an evidence-based professional because when you encounter other articles with similar features, you will know how to use the information in your decision making.

The constraint-induced therapy articles you have read in this unit provide an opportunity to learn about other characteristics of articles. In the Methods section, Klingels et al. (2013) has standard headings, while Kitago et al. (2013) uses many subheadings to alert the reader to the components (e.g., participants, measures). This difference is likely related to the format and traditions of these journals. Although subheadings are user friendly for readers, they take up precious space. How does this difference affect you as a consumer of the studies?

UNDERSTAND DATA IN TABLES AND FIGURES

The Kitago et al. (2013) article contains tables and figures that help illustrate their findings for the reader. These authors provide information about their findings in three ways. First, they provide a summary of the baseline scores for their patients in Table 2. This is a common type of table for a study like this. Second, they report in the text which comparisons are significant. Third, they take some of the information and graph it for you in the figures. Let's use Figure 2 as an example. This figure shows visually the comparisons of the means and error bars of the ARAT totals. These are called a box and whisker plot; the "whiskers" extend to show the error range. The third box and whisker plot corresponds to the post-treatment scores.

If you now refer to the text (pp. 103-104), you will see that they report a significant difference between the two pretreatment and the post-treatment testing periods. The graph illustrates the magnitude of this change (i.e., comparing the first and second box and whisker plots to the third one on Figure 2A).

Many authors only report the numbers and significance without the graph. Now that you see this example, you can always make a graph like this for yourself using data from any article (using the mean and standard deviation) if a figure would help you see the comparison better.

Evidence Detective Tip

When unsure about the comparisons being made,
graph the means and standard deviations for the groups into make a visual image
reflecting the similarities or differences between the groups.

Activity 8-7
Practice With Your Study Partners

Work with your study partners to examine Table 2 (Klingels et al., 2013). Find the text that is associated with Table 2. Can you find the same *p* values that are mentioned in both the text and the Table? See if you can follow across the appropriate rows in Table 2 as the authors describe the findings for the primary outcome.

Now let's look at Figure 2 (Klingels et al., 2013). Figure 2 shows the prognostic factors associated with the outcomes from the study. Specifically, they found "a significant interaction…" What does this mean? When research studies are conducted, we hope that the only thing that leads to change (if any) in our study participants is the intervention. However, other things may influence whether or not or how much changes study participants experience. It this case, as shown in Figure 2A, age played a role in the outcome the children experienced. Younger children (aged 4.5 to 8 years) in both groups got better but older children (aged 8 to 12 years) only got better if they were in the m-CIMT+IT group. Using what you just learned from Figure 2A, describe what's going in Figure 2B. What is the "prognostic factor" at play here? How did it influence the outcomes for different groups? What do the different colors in Figure 2B mean?

Activity 8-8
Practice With Your Study Partners

Discuss which graphing strategy you like the most or least. Which article provided the clearest link between the numeric data and the illustrations? What was unclear? What suggestions would you make to improve one or all of these articles?

UNDERSTANDING FAMILIAR MEASURES

The Kitago et al. (2013) study used a measure that may not be familiar to readers. The authors give readers references for learning more about the measure, and then they provide an informative summary so readers can evaluate their findings. They provide the subdomains of the measure. Further, the authors use kinematic measures that are usually only used in laboratory settings but have begun to be used in clinical practice. They provide examples of the tasks that the children have to complete. This strategy enables readers to imagine what happened in the study and then decide whether the measure would be applicable to a practice population (i.e., Could the children I serve do these tasks? What would they look like when doing them?).

LEARN MORE ABOUT INTERVENTIONS

Each of these studies examined the effectiveness of constraint-induced therapy. However, they did not use exactly the same procedures for their interventions.

Evidence Detective Tip

Sometimes the measures reported in studies would be useful in your practice.

Activity 8-9
Compare Features of Interventions

Worksheet: Compare Intervention Programs

Meet with your study partners to compare and contrast the features of the intervention program for the three studies. One aspect has been added to the worksheet to get you started; complete the worksheet to plan for your meeting. After your complete your discussion of the similarities and differences, write a summary statement that includes the best intervention features for an effective intervention program based on these studies.

Activity 8-10
Know What the Public Might Know

The topic of constraint-induced therapy has gotten a lot of public attention, so you will be able to find newspaper and magazine articles that report on the research for the public. Find an article that journalistically reports on the findings of a research article and share it with your study partners. Consider the following issues in your discussion.

Sometimes public press articles do not use person-first language.

- Does your article use negative connotations that would be unacceptable in professional literature (e.g., saying "stroke victims" has two negative features: first, saying stroke as the initial word, which defines the person as a disability rather than as a person, and second, saying victim, which presumes that the experience of having a stroke is automatically negative)?

- What are the differences between what actual professional authors say about their findings and what journalists say about the findings?

- In what ways might the public be served by this journalist report?

- In what ways might the public be misled by this journalist report?

- How do science and evidence advance with public articles such as this one?

Activity 8-11
Develop Take-Home Messages

Worksheet: Create Take-Home Messages

The final step in the analysis process for evidence-based practice is to summarize the findings for those who need to use the ideas to improve their practices. Professionals want clear, easy-to-understand guidelines about what to do. We will call these summaries "Take-Home Messages" to remind ourselves to use understandable language. You will need to consider Take-Home Messages for your colleagues (within your discipline and from other disciplines), family members, other care providers, and those receiving your care.

Select two constituent groups as the focus of your attention and create some Take-Home Messages for them. Pretend that the articles you read were the **definitive** articles on the topic. Use the worksheet to summarize your work.

When considering what you are going to write, think about these questions:

- What would you say to colleagues about how they might need to change their practices to gain the optimal benefit?
- What would you say to your team regarding the articles' findings based on the articles you have read?
- How would you extrapolate information from these articles to develop hypotheses for populations other than the ones that were studied?

SUMMARY

In this unit, you learned about constraint-induced therapy. Although all the studies addressed this topic, they each had individualized ways of applying the concept to their interventions. These distinctions are important to detect in evidence-based practice. Professionals have to make decisions about how much, how long, etc., every day.

Examining Evidence Related to Upper Extremity Fractures

During this unit, you will explore some evidence about upper extremity fractures. Both articles include a rehabilitation team approach to treatment and involve occupational therapists partnering with those from other disciplines. Though this topic may seem very nuanced and specific, it includes good examples of study designs. The findings from the articles also the value of introducing rehabilitation very early after surgery. The discussion sections of each article highlight the importance of the interdisciplinary team. The authors also present their findings only in tables. This gives us a chance to practice graphing data into a format that makes more sense when we consider how much of an impact the intervention can have for our clients.

When you complete the work for this unit, you will have the following skills and competencies:

- Articulating how to find other articles that would contribute to your knowledge about this topic
- Articulating the distinct value of occupational therapy as a part of an interdisciplinary team
- Creating graphs and figures from data presented in a table
- Constructing Take-Home Messages for various constituents so they can quickly understand what the literature says about this topic

You will be reviewing articles, creating summaries for comparison and contrast, gaining insights from your study partners, creating graphs of data from the articles, and creating Take-Home Messages for constituent groups.

Activity 9-1
Read the Literature

We will consider two articles for this unit. Read both articles, focusing on the methods and the results. It is not necessary to understand all the background for the study.

Dunn, W., & Proffitt, R. *Bringing Evidence Into Everyday Practice: Practical Strategies for Health Care Professionals, Second Edition* (pp. 65-73). © 2024 Taylor & Francis Group.

Content warning: The He et al. (2021) article has images on p. 6 of the external fixation during surgery.

Filipova, V., Lonzaric, D., & Papez, B. J. (2015). *Efficacy of combined physical and occupational therapy in patients with conservatively treated distal radius fracture: Randomized controlled trial.* Central European Journal of Medicine, 127(Suppl. 5), S282-S287. https://doi.org/10.1007/s00508-015-0812-9

He, M., Wang, Q., Zhao, J., & Wang, Y. (2021). *Efficacy of ultra-early rehabilitation on elbow function after Slongo's external fixation for supracondylar humeral fractures in older children and adolescents.* Journal of Orthopedic Surgery and Research, 16(520), e1-e7. https://doi.org/10.1186/s13018-021-02671-4

Activity 9-2
Summarize Methods and Results
Worksheet: Summarize the Characteristics of a Research Article

Create a summary table using the worksheet for these articles. Though the articles use different approaches and populations, you will be able to see overlaps in the approaches and findings.

Summary tables show readers the most important aspects of studies. Locate a summary article in an area of your interest and see how its tables are organized. You can use your findings to help you make your own summary table. Make your summary table work for your learning and information needs.

LOOKING FOR PATTERNS AND THEMES

First, look for similarities and differences in the structures of the studies.

- Did they study the same populations?
- Did they use similar settings?
- Were the designs similar?
- How did the measures compare to each other?

The answers to these questions can help you understand differences in findings. For example, if one study says an intervention worked and another study says it did not, you will need to examine these other factors to see what might have contributed to the differences. In these studies, one intervention lasted for 6 months while the other intervention lasted for 4 weeks; if there are differences in the findings, we might hypothesize about the influence of these time periods on the outcomes reported.

Now, think about the topic.

- What happened to your thinking from before and after reading the articles?
- How did your ideas change?
- Have you observed that professionals have incorporated these findings into their practices?
- Are you going to do anything differently now that you have read these studies?

These questions enable you to examine how the findings affected yours and others' thinking about practice. A great study that professionals are skeptical about will not have an impact on the practices. As professionals we need to understand the reasons why people may or may not adopt a strategy that has been shown effective through a research study.

⁙⁙⁙⁙⁙⁙⁙⁙⁙⁙⁙⁙⁙⁙⁙⁙⁙⁙⁙⁙⁙⁙⁙⁙⁙⁙⁙⁙⁙⁙⁙⁙⁙⁙⁙⁙⁙⁙⁙

Activity 9-3
Recognize Strengths and Limitations

Worksheet: Identify Answerable and Unanswerable Questions

All research articles make a contribution and have limitations. Perhaps a group of articles is only about one age group and diagnosis—then we are not sure whether we can apply their findings to other age groups and other diagnoses. There will always be practice questions that can and cannot be answered by the available research. Sometimes researchers conduct studies about what can be answered, but that does not mean that studies reflect the only important topics for practice. Perhaps there are no measures to find out the answer to an important practice question. It might be that a population is so heterogeneous that it is hard to detect changes or discover who would or would not profit from an intervention. In practice, there will always be answerable and unanswerable questions. Advances in measurement, technology, and knowledge make more questions answerable.

Considering this group of articles, complete the worksheet about the answerable and unanswerable questions for practice.

Activity 9-4
Handle Anomalous Data

Worksheet: Reactions to New Data

The findings from these articles may challenge some of your current beliefs. Refer to your Executive Summary (see Sidebar 2-1) of the Chinn and Brewer (1993) article to decide where your reactions to the article findings are occurring. Bring these issues up with your study partners.

Activity 9-5
Expand the Evidence

Obtain another article (i.e., in the past 5 years) that adds information to your understanding about this topic. Add this citation, etc., to your summary worksheet. Make copies of your article for your study partners.

Activity 9-6
Group Discussion

Meet with your study partners and discuss your findings and reactions to the articles. Add your unique information to the discussion from the article you are contributing on the topic. Refine your notes based on your discussion.

EXTENDING KNOWLEDGE ABOUT METHODS AND RESULTS

Every set of articles reflects an overall topic. Additionally, each article illustrates some unique features of studies and ways to report the methods and findings. By examining some aspects of each study, you will accumulate knowledge about designs and statistics while learning more about the evidence. This process will build your capacity as an evidence-based professional because when you encounter other articles with similar features, you will know how to use the information in your decision making.

The upper extremity fracture articles in this unit provide an opportunity to learn about other characteristics of articles. These two studies used different statistical analyses, time frames, and measured different aspects of recovery and function in different ways. Some professionals might be more familiar with one approach or measure, making that article's findings more inviting to their practice. Some professionals in hospital-based settings might already have existing rehabilitation programs, but do not have a good relationship with the surgeons; if this is the case, the early rehabilitation intervention might not be as appealing or feasible.

Activity 9-7
Make Graphs From Tables

The tables in both of these studies are very detailed and provide the reader with a comprehensive view of their findings. This can be overwhelming to readers who are either novices to the topic or those who are unfamiliar with the statistical procedures. We will examine portions of the tables here so you can become more familiar with how to read and make use of their data for these and other studies.

We looked at data in the constraint-induced therapy articles in Unit 8 and how graphs of the data could increase understanding about the comparisons. In these upper extremity fracture articles, the authors use only tables and make notations on the tables indicating what comparisons are significantly different. The Filipova et al. (2015) article contains three different tables with several columns in each, and the He et al. (2021) article contains four tables with a lot of comparisons between groups. Whew! This is a lot of information to digest.

Both articles report data on their study participants in Table 1. The He et al. (2021) article includes more details about the study participants. Table 1 in the He et al. (2021) article has a third column with p values. Why would the authors want to report p values in this table if these data are from **before** the intervention happened? Many researchers that use randomized study designs will use statistical tests to compare the two groups at baseline. This helps them confirm that randomization worked! Researchers want to ensure that the two groups are balanced across the demographic and clinical characteristics. Look at the *p* values in Table 1 of the He et al. (2021) article. Are there any variables that are different between the two groups?

The next few tables in each article report the main findings. Both articles include mean values for the two groups at multiple time points. The He et al. (2021) article uses mean and standard deviations in Table 2 to report on the primary outcomes. The Filipova et al. (2015) article reports data using mean, 95% confidence interval, and median. All are commonly used in reporting data. A 95% confidence interval gives us an understanding of the range of values. The standard deviation gives us an understanding of the variability or "spread" of the data (e.g., a short and squat bell curve or a tall, tightly compressed bell curve).

As we look at the *p* values in Table 2 of the He et al. (2021) article, we notice that there are several that are less than the commonly used .05 cutoff. The authors state on p. 3 that *p* < .05 was considered to be statistically significant. However, we have to look at the footnotes of the table to help us understand which *p* values are linked to which comparison of groups. This is when a well-made graph can provide instant clarity on differences within and between groups.

Graphs can also help us understand the magnitude of difference in comparisons. A *p* value of .007 means that this difference would be in error less than 1 in 7,000 times. For most people, this would be convincing. With a difference of this magnitude, you might expect that the two groups are radically different. Let's graph the data to see what *p* = .007 looks like in this case. Using the data from Table 2, Row 1 (flexion in affected side, degrees), Figure 9-1 is a graph of that comparison along with the other two comparisons. The asterisks indicate comparisons that are statistically significant. Looking at their graph, we can clearly see that there were differences at 3 months and 6 months between the two groups. We can also see that for the rehabilitation group, there were statistically significant differences from 3 to 6 months.

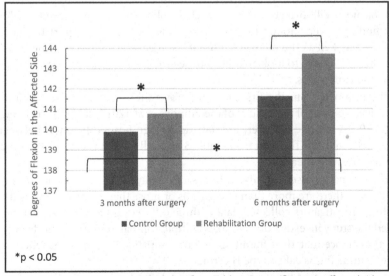

Figure 9-1. Graph of He et al. (2021) data from Table 2, Row 1 (flexion in affected side, degrees). The asterisks indicate comparisons that are statistically significant.

From the data we see that there was an increase of just about 3 degrees of elbow flexion for the rehabilitation group and slightly less for the control group. This is an additional way to consider the size of the difference; when a study is about your interest area, you will have a better idea whether this much change matters.

An evidence-based professional must not only consider the statistical significance of a comparison, but must also consider the effect size of the difference. The effect size can be calculated several ways and tells us the magnitude of the difference between two conditions (Portney & Watkins, 2009). For our type of test (independent samples t-test), we can use the difference in the means divided by the pooled standard deviation. For the comparison between the groups at 3 months, the effect size is 0.21. This is a small effect size, as we might expect. A difference of 3 degrees of elbow flexion is not much! In a later unit on meta-analyses, we will consider the average effect size across a group of studies. Tickle-Degnen (2001), discussed in Unit 10, also provides a helpful discussion about application of effect size to evidence-based practice.

Activity 9-8
Practice With Your Study Partners

Work with your study partners to create graphs for the other variables in Table 2 of the He et al. (2021) article. Discuss whether you think that the statistically significant changes matter in actual practice. Make graphs of the data from Tables 3 and 4. Lastly, make a graph of the data from the last row of Table 1. The time (in weeks) to range of motion required for activities of daily living (ROM-ADL) is likely more meaningful for occupational therapy practitioners. Discuss with your study partners what you consider to be meaningful change. How might the study participants feel with the changes shown in the tables? If these amounts seem inadequate, what amount would?

Now let's look at the Filipova et al. (2015) article's tables. These authors used a different strategy to report their findings, even though they are also using tables. They report the means and 95% confidence intervals as well as the median for all of the measures in Table 2. There are no p values included in this table. We have to look at Table 3 to see the p values for the comparisons within and between groups and timepoints.

We used the numbers from the first and third rows (Table 2, Wrist Flexion and Hand Grip Strength, respectively, p. S284 of the article) of the Filipova et al. (2015) table to create Figure 9-2. The asterisks in Figure 9-2A indicate that there are statistically significant differences between the groups in grip strength at T2 and T3. The data from Table 3 also tell us that there is an interaction of time and therapy. What does this mean?

The type of statistical test used for this study was a two-way mixed analysis of variance (ANOVA). ANOVA is used when there are more than two groups or more than two time points in the study. In this case, the study investigators collected data at three different time points across the two groups. ANOVA allowed the study investigators to make multiple comparisons across and within the groups and minimize the chance that they found something statistically significant when there actually wasn't anything to find. This is called type II error.

In Figure 9-2B we see that both groups improved, but there were no differences between the groups. There was an effect of time but no effect of group (or treatment). Similarly, in Figure 9-2A, we see that both groups did improve. What is different is that Group B (PT + FOT) got even better than Group A (PT) over time. This simultaneous effect of both therapy and time is called an interaction effect.

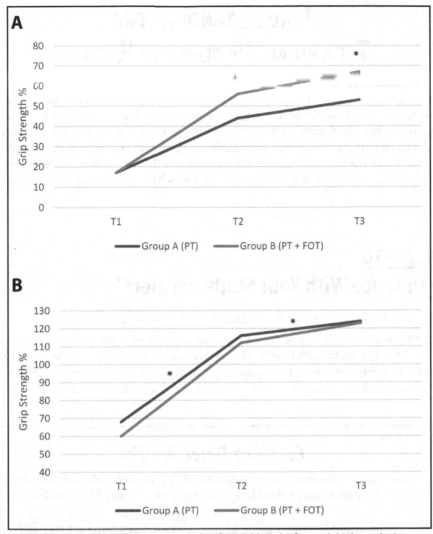

Figure 9-2. Graph of Filopova et al. (2015) data from Table 2, the first and third rows (wrist flexion and hand grip strength, respectively). (A) indicates that there are statistically significant differences between the groups in grip strength at T2 and T3. (B) indicates that both groups improved, but there were no differences between the groups.

<u>Activity 9-9</u>
Practice With Your Study Partners

Work with your study partners to graph the other variables in Table 2 and interpret what you see. Does your interpretation match the *p* values in Table 3?

UNDERSTANDING THE
TECHNICAL WORDING IN RESULTS

Another challenge for professionals looking for evidence is making sense of the technical reporting of results in the text of articles. Although we cannot be experts at all statistics, it is helpful to know how to acquire a basic understanding of the way researchers report their findings. Knowing this, when you peruse the Results sections of an article, you can make your own decisions about the study findings. You can decide whether you agree or disagree with the authors' interpretations (in the Discussion section). Researchers are expected to report only the facts in the Results sections; whereas researchers have more latitude in the Discussion section, where they are explaining what they think the data mean.

Activity 9-10
More Practice With Your Study Partners

Worksheet: Analyze the Results Section of an Article

We have filled in the first column of the worksheet with excerpts from the Results section of Filipova et al. (2015). Meet with your study partners to review the Results section. Use Portney (2020), or another research design and statistics text, to help you interpret the excerpts. Write in your own words what each excerpt means in the second column of the worksheet.

Evidence Detective Tip

Sometimes comparisons can be statistically significant and yet reflect changes
that are small when considering the person's everyday life behavior.

Look at the actual amount of change in a behavior and ask yourself
whether that amount of change would be noticeable in your practice and
whether it is likely to contribute to improved satisfaction or participation.

This is what "effect size" calculations will tell you when they are reported in studies.

Activity 9-11
Develop Take-Home Messages

Worksheet: Create Take-Home Messages

The final step in the analysis process for evidence-based practice is to summarize the findings for those who need to use the ideas to improve their practices. Professionals want clear, easy-to-understand guidelines about what to do. We will call these summaries "Take-Home Messages" to remind ourselves to use understandable language. You will need to consider Take-Home Messages for your colleagues (within your discipline and from other disciplines), family members, other care providers, and those receiving your care.

Select two constituent groups as the focus of your attention and create some Take-Home Messages for them. Pretend that the articles you read were the **definitive** articles on the topic. Use the worksheet to summarize your work.

When considering what you are going to write, think about these questions:

- What would you say to colleagues about how they might need to change their practices to gain the optimal benefit?
- What would you say to your team regarding the articles' findings based on the articles you have read?
- How would you extrapolate information from these articles to develop hypotheses for other populations than the ones that were studied?

SUMMARY

In this unit you examined research related to upper extremity fractures. You compared the various strategies used in the interventions and the outcomes associated with those strategies. You got practice understanding and graphing results from tables, and then deciding what the results mean for clinical practice. These skills will be useful in interpreting findings from a variety of articles.

Expanding Your Knowledge and Skills for Evidence-Based Practice

There are additional resources available to support evidence-based practice. Scholars conduct formal reviews of the literature so you can have summaries and recommendations from others. Emerging ideas in professional practice often don't have evidence, so you need to have other strategies for evaluating these ideas. Professionals also need to collect their own data within their practices to verify the effectiveness of any evidence, emerging or established. Lastly, communicating evidence to consumers and stakeholders is an important component of the evidence-based practice triad.

Understanding Summary and Meta-Analysis Articles

During this unit, you will explore evidence from articles that summarize a body of literature for us. In addition to individual studies, you can get good information for your evidence-based practice from summary articles that review all the literature available on a specific topic.

Summary articles are helpful because you can get a lot of research findings from one source. The author has synthesized findings for you, and so you can get a bigger picture more efficiently. You can find summary articles in typical professional library sources and on some specialized websites on the internet (e.g., the Cochrane Collaboration).

When you complete the work for this unit, you will have the following skills and competencies:

- Being familiar with the format of summary articles and what they tell us about an area of practice
- Understanding the special characteristics of meta-analyses as summary articles
- Knowing how to access websites that provide summary material to guide evidence-based practice
- Constructing best practice tips for colleagues from a summary article to guide practice decisions
- Constructing Take-Home Messages for various constituents so they understand quickly what the literature says about the topic

You will be reviewing articles, analyzing the process of article selection, gaining insights from your study partners, and creating Take-Home Messages for constituent groups.

The Portney (2020) text provides a guide in Chapter 37 to help you with this material. We will examine a meta-analysis article, a scoping review article, and one summary article in this unit.

Dunn, W., & Proffitt, R. *Bringing Evidence Into Everyday Practice: Practical Strategies for Health Care Professionals, Second Edition* (pp. 77-87). © 2024 Taylor & Francis Group.

INTRODUCTION TO USE OF META-ANALYSIS

A meta-analysis is a special type of summary information article. It analyzes the findings of a whole set of studies using specialized statistical procedures. Although research and evidence-based practice texts explain what a meta-analysis is and how to construct and understand the analysis, professionals also need to understand how to **use** the valuable summary information from a meta-analysis to guide their practice decisions. Tickle-Degnen (2001) provides a very helpful discussion for professionals.

> Tickle-Degnen, L. (2001). From the general to the specific: Using meta-analytic reports in clinical decision making. Evaluation and the Health Professions, 24(3), 308-326. https://doi.org/10.1177/01632780122034939

She explains that professionals must consider whether the information in the meta-analysis actually applies to the person(s) in their practice. First, professionals must determine whether the characteristics of the research participants match the characteristics of the persons being served; if they don't match, we must consider whether the outcomes would generalize to our particular client. Second, professionals must determine which research participants responded to which aspects of the interventions; we are more at risk if we apply an intervention that was effective overall but not with the type of person being served. Tickle-Degnen (2001) applies findings of a study about exercise poststroke to a particular individual, Mrs. Jones. We will use a more recent meta-analysis here—use the Tickle-Degnen article to guide your work on the meta-analysis. Let's apply the information from the text and article readings to a portion of a meta-analysis so we can practice.

ANALYSIS OF A META-ANALYSIS

Let's study the components of a meta-analysis. You will need to use excerpts from the following study here within this unit. Please obtain the full study so you can review the full work with your study partners.

> Ikiugu, M. N., Nissen, R. M., Bellar, C., Maassen, A., & Van Peursem, K. (2017). Clinical effectiveness of occupational therapy in mental health: A meta-analysis. American Journal of Occupational Therapy, 71(5), 7105100020p1-7105100020p10. https://doi.org/10.5014/ajot.2017.024588

As you have been learning, the abstract provides an overview of the work. Following the format prescribed by this journal, the authors provide the readers with four subheadings:

1. Objective
2. Method
3. Results
4. Conclusion

Objective

Ikiugu et al. (2017) succinctly tell what their goal was for the study. Some authors write a statement of purpose, while other authors use a question format to tell readers what they are studying.

Activity 10-1
Dissect the Abstract

Write the abstract (see Sidebar 10-1) in your own words since these authors related the outcome of the study, change it to a question and put it into your own words.

Sidebar 10-1
Case Study: Sarah

Sarah is a 73-year-old woman who participates in a community mental health program in her community. She loves to garden, wants to grocery shop on her own, and wants to cook. The team needs to decide how they will partner with Sarah to design a plan to meet her goals.

Now compare with your study partners. What did you miss? What did you highlight compared to others?

This abstract gives the reader an overview about how the authors picked articles they would analyze, the statistical procedures they used, the outcomes that were measured, and the outcomes of their analysis. From this part of the abstract, readers learn about the study and can get a sense about whether this meta-analysis would be applicable to their practices.

The authors summarize the parameters of their findings at the end of the summary. These are the findings that you can use to guide your practice based on the evidence.

Examine the Methods

In this article, you have to look inside the paper itself to find out the specific methods they used to select studies for their meta-analysis. Under the heading "Research Design" they tell you whose procedures they will follow (Borenstein et al., 2009; Portney & Watkins, 2009) and provide you with a rationale for their selection. Then they tell you how they defined "occupational performance" and "well-being," the variables of interest in this study.

One of the most important aspects of a meta-analysis is the selection of search criteria. The words a researcher selects will determine which articles get included or excluded. This is similar to selecting which people get into a study (e.g., only adults with a stroke within the last 2 years).

Activity 10-2
Find the Search Terms

Work with your study partners to make a comprehensive list of search terms.

Look through the method section of Ikiugu et al. (2017) and make a list of key words the authors used to conduct their search. You will have to consider how they found "occupational performance" and "well-being" studies, how they determined whether there was a theoretical foundation (one of their criteria), what types of studies they allowed, what data had to be included in the study (so they could conduct the meta-analysis), and who they accepted as participants.

Find one study that is more recent (i.e., 2018 or newer) that would meet all these criteria. Share these with your study partners and tell them how your study meets all the criteria.

Study the Results

Now let's look at a portion of the results of this study.

Identify Eligible Studies for the Meta-Analysis

One of the most challenging aspects of meta-analyses is the selection of the studies to be included. In this study, the authors set some initial criteria and then began looking for articles in professional databases. The authors considered 6,534 citations before selecting the 11 that they analyzed. They used a systematic process for making decisions about which studies to include, as you saw in the prior activity.

The authors provide a flow chart illustrating the process these authors used to go from 6,534 studies to 11 studies for their meta-analysis. This process will help you understand how to make systematic decisions for yourself when selecting studies to review in your practice.

Activity 10-3
Analyze the Flow Chart of Article Selection

Look at the flow chart on their Figure 1.

Work with your study partners to identify what questions the authors asked themselves at each step in the flow chart.

- How did they go from 6,534 to 94 studies?
- What questions got them from 94 to 75 studies?
- What did they exclude to get from 75 to the final 11 studies?

Looking carefully at a flow chart such as this helps you understand the thinking process that you will need to use to find appropriate studies in your practice.

Activity 10-4
Practice Making Flow Charts for Yourself

With this little bit of practice, what are some questions and criteria you might include in a sorting process for your practice? Create a draft of the decision process you might use for a question in a practice area of interest to you.

Share your ideas with your study partners. Critique each other's plans so you can use this draft when you get into your fieldwork and first job.

Look at the Graphs in the Results

The results section of this article is hard to read, especially if you are new to reading summary review studies. There is a lot of technical information to illustrate to a more advanced reader that the authors used appropriate procedures systematically. There are some interesting characteristics of these results. Let's look at them together.

Activity 10-5
Walk Through the Graphs and Findings Together

Work as a class or with study partners to examine the findings together. Here are some guiding statements to help you along.

First, it is easy to notice the Funnel graphs in Figures 2 and 3. These graphs are showing the reader how homogeneous (alike) the study findings were. In the text, the authors tell us that they found some of their 11 studies to be heterogeneous (different) from the others. There were 7 studies that addressed occupational performance, and 7 studies that addressed well-being. (Since there were 11 studies in total, this means that a few studies addressed both outcomes.)

The authors did not provide much information about the figures on their actual figures. This makes it hard to interpret the figures without wading through the text; they could have provided more description and labels on the graphs to make them easier to review independently from the text. Figure 2 illustrates the range of differences in the studies about occupational performance. Figure 3 illustrates the range of differences in the studies about well-being.

Let's look at Figure 3. You can see that two of the dots are solid, while five of the dots are open. They are showing you the two weakest studies (solid dots) in comparison to the five stronger studies (open dots). You can see that if we consider all seven studies there is a large amount of variability from the bottom study (about -0.5 standardized differences in means) to the top study (about 1.3 standardized differences in means). A standardized difference in means is a calculation that equates all the means across studies to make comparison easier to see.

Draw a horizontal line from the lowest to highest dot so you can see the range.

With all the variability you see in Figure 3, it is hard to make conclusions about the well-being outcome. So the authors used a procedure to exclude the bottom two studies. You can see that when you exclude these two studies, the range is much smaller (i.e., from about 0.4 to 1.3 standardized differences in means).

Now draw a horizontal line from the lowest to highest OPEN dot so you can see the range.

With more homogeneity, it is easier for the authors to draw conclusions about what theories and interventions were the most helpful for a well-being outcome. Don't you want to know which study is represented by the highest dot? It piques our curiosity; what was distinct about this study? Perhaps the participants were younger, or perhaps they used a particular theory and approach that the others did not. It sure looks like something important happened in that study.

Activity 10-6
Critique the Authors' Ideas

Meet with your study partners to dissect some of the results. We will just select one area to critique to learn how to think this way. You can apply this strategy to other parts of this article, and to other articles you read as well.

Just under Figure 2 in the article, the authors state:

Analysis for moderators revealed that much of the variability could be attributed to two outlier studies ($n = 102$) in which unspecified client-centered theory and the psychodynamic model were used to guide intervention strategies. A small effect of intervention was found, based on unspecified client-centered principles, on well-being that favored the control group ... (p. 5)

- What does this passage mean? Restate it to each other in your own words.
- The authors talk about "unspecified client-centered theory," what do you think they mean by this? How did their inclusion criteria account for "unspecified client-centered theory?" What do you think their rationale was for including studies with this theoretical basis? How could the authors have provided readers with more information to increase clarity?
- What bias might be present with their decision-making process? What actions could guard against possible bias?

Discussion of the Discussion

As you have learned, the Discussion section of an article expands the ideas from the study by providing interpretation and hypotheses about why the findings turned out the way they did. Read the Ikiugu et al. (2017) discussion to learn what the authors think about the details of their findings.

Activity 10-7
Identify Take-Home Messages From the Authors

Worksheet: Create Take-Home Messages

The authors looked at the details of the studies and have several insights to offer the readers. List the things they suggest are the Take-Home Messages from their study using the worksheet we have been using throughout this workbook. For the rationale component, find a quote from the study. Compare your list with your study partners. What did you miss? What did you have that others missed?

Activity 10-8
Limitations of the Study

The discussion also describes the limitations of the study. This is expected from editors so authors take responsibility for what they could and could not accomplish in their current study. This is like the answerable and unanswerable questions worksheet we have been using. Because this is a meta-analysis, the authors point out limitations in the articles available to them for their study.

Meet with your study partners and discuss what recommendations you would make to future researchers to address the limitations.

What Does This Study Mean for Your Practice?

Activity 10-9
Apply Findings to Practice

This paper includes implications for occupational therapy. Meet with your study partners and discuss the authors' recommendations.

- Discuss what all quality services for people with mental illness need to address.
- Discuss how documentation might change based on the authors' recommendations.
- Outline a best practice plan for a community mental health program based on these implications.

Activity 10-10
Apply Findings to a Specific Practice Situation

Worksheet: Apply Evidence to a Specific Situation

The general findings of a meta-analysis are not always applicable to a specific person in your practice. Let's practice applying findings to a specific situation.

Read Sarah's case (see Sidebar 10-1). Pretend that you and your study partners are the community mental health team serving Sarah. Considering the findings of the Ikiugu et al. (2017) article, what will your plans be for Sarah's program? Complete the worksheet with your team.

When we look at the articles in the Ikiugu et al. (2017) meta-analysis, we see that some articles contain research participants who are like Sarah. None of the studies look at the particular long-term outcomes Sarah is after, but the team therapists decide that they will look at the findings and discuss what to do.

When looking at the articles that apply to Sarah, the team sees that some of them are not very strong studies according to the article's methodology analysis, and the weaker studies have questionable effect sizes as well (i.e., the magnitude of the difference between intervention and control groups is small). The stronger studies use different theoretical approaches, so the team will have to discuss the best approach with Sarah.

Using Scoping Review Articles

Another way to summarize the literature is with a scoping review. Scoping reviews are more descriptive and exploratory, and are a great choice when there is emerging research literature in an area of interest rather than a plethora of experimental studies. Scoping reviews provide a broad view of the landscape in a particular area and indicate directions for future work. They are perfect choices for many topics in occupational therapy literature. Here are some examples from occupational therapy to give you a sense of the possibilities.

Bushby, K., Chan, J., Druif, S., Ho, K., & Kinsella, E. A. (2015). *Ethical tensions in occupational therapy practice: A scoping review.* British Journal of Occupational Therapy, *78(4), 212-221.* https://doi.org/10.1177/0308022614564770

Conn, A., Bourke, N., James, C., & Haracz, K. (2019). *Occupational therapy intervention addressing weight gain and obesity in people with severe mental illness: A scoping review.* Australian Occupational Therapy Journal, *66(4), 446-457.* https://doi.org/10.1111/1440-1630.12575

Hand, C., Law, M., & McColl, M. A. (2011). *Occupational therapy interventions for chronic diseases: A scoping review.* American Journal of Occupational Therapy, *65(4), 428-436.* https://doi.org/10.5014/ajot.2011.002071

Lal, S., Jarus, T., & Suto, M. J. (2012). *A scoping review of the photovoice method: Implications for occupational therapy research.* Canadian Journal of Occupational Therapy, *79(3), 181-190.* https://doi.org/10.2182/cjot.2012.79.3.8

Truong, V., & Hodgetts, S. (2017). *An exploration of teacher perceptions toward occupational therapy and occupational therapy practices: A scoping review.* Journal of Occupational Therapy, Schools, & Early Intervention, *10(2), 121-136.* https://doi.org/10.1080/19411243.2017.1304840

Wallis, A., Meredith, P., & Stanley, M. (2020). *Cancer care and occupational therapy: A scoping review.* Australian Occupational Therapy Journal, *67(2), 172-194.* https://doi.org/10.1111/1440-1630.12633

Let's look more closely at Conn et al. (2019). Obtain the article so you can follow along as we look at their methods and results.

Activity 10-11
Review the Flow Chart

Figure 1 contains a similar flow chart as we saw in the meta-analysis article (Ikiugu et al., 2017). Open both articles to compare them. Meet with your study partners to identify the similarities and differences.

- What is the same about the two flow charts?
- What is distinct about each flow chart? How do these distinctions inform you about the different types of summary articles (i.e., meta-analysis vs. scoping review)?
- What is the meaning of Ikiugu et al. (2017) starting out with more than 6,000 articles and the Conn et al. (2019) article starting out with 43 articles?

Activity 10-12
Identify Search Parameters

Worksheet: Identify Search Parameters in a Summary Study

Use the worksheet to identify the search parameters for the Conn et al. (2019) scoping review. You will see in this study that the authors also included explicit exclusion criteria. How does this help refine the search? Discuss your ideas with your study partners.

EXPLORING THEMATIC ANALYSIS

The Conn et al. (2019) article provides a summary table (Table 1) of the selected articles. You will see that this table is similar to the Summarize the Characteristics of a Research Article worksheet you have been using throughout this text. Now that you are relying on the authors to provide you with details, it is less work for you, but take note of how helpful this table is for you now that you have completed some of these tables yourself. The format is familiar, you know what to focus on and what to expect, and you probably can get to key information more readily. All readers are grateful for details such as these, and your experience makes this table more accessible for you.

Because this is a scoping review, the authors conducted a thematic analysis to discover common ideas across the studies. There is text describing their themes under the Results, and they provide readers with a summary in their Table 2. These authors also focus on theoretical supports and show how their themes line up with the PEOP model in the last column.

Activity 10-13
Apply Findings to a Specific Practice Situation

Worksheet: Apply Evidence to a Specific Situation

The general findings of a meta-analysis are not always applicable to a specific person in your practice. Let's practice applying findings to a specific situation.

Read Sarah's case (see Sidebar 10-1) again, with the additional idea that obesity is interfering with Sarah meeting her goals. Pretend that you and your study partners are the community mental health team serving Sarah. Considering the findings of the Conn et al. (2019) article, what will your plans be for Sarah's program? Complete the worksheet with your team.

Since there are many themes and subthemes, select one category as the focus of your attention. Read the authors' descriptions of that theme/subtheme as the background for your plans.

ANALYSIS OF A SUMMARY ARTICLE

Summary or review papers examine a set of articles about a particular topic, just as meta-analyses do. The difference is that summary articles do not have the same requirements for searching and analyzing the findings (i.e., there are more restrictions in a meta-analysis). Please obtain the full study of Spencer et al. (2018) so you can follow along with this discussion.

Spencer, B., Sherman, L., Nielsen, S., & Thormodson, K. (2018). Effectiveness of occupational therapy interventions for students with mental illness transitioning to higher education: A systematic review. Occupational Therapy in Mental Health, 34(2), 151-164. https://doi.org/10.1080/0164212X.2017.1380559

You will notice several structural differences in this article when we compare it to the Ikiugu et al. (2017) and Conn et al. (2019) articles.

Activity 10-14
Compare and Contrast Article Formats

Meet with your study partners and compile a list of similarities of the formats of the three articles.

- What is common across all the articles?
- What is distinct about each article? How does this distinction reflect the summary approach (i.e., meta-analysis, scoping, summary review)?

EXAMINE THE PURPOSE OF THE ARTICLE

The Spencer et al. (2018) authors state a purpose and research questions for their study. Discuss in class which one is more meaningful for you, and provide a rationale.

Activity 10-15
Review the Structure of This Review

Meet in class or with your study partners to discuss the structure of this review article.

The Spencer et al. (2018) article employs some different strategies for presenting the research plan. First, they provide a Population Intervention Comparison Outcome (PICO) table to outline their plan, which provides definitions of terms of interest. How is this helpful to the readers? Who might find this PICO table daunting, and how could we adapt the information for different types of cognitive strategies?

Second, Spencer et al. (2018) provides a table (Table 2) listing the search terms. In the prior articles, you had to figure out what the search terms were likely to be based on the authors' descriptions. How could this table be useful to you when using this study in your practice setting?

Figure 1 provides the flow chart for decision making. Follow their decision process to see how they got from 4,040 articles to the 7 articles they accepted into their review. Then, pause for a moment, and appreciate what these authors (and the prior authors) did to save you so much time. How long do you think it took to review 4,040 articles and make systematic decisions based on their inclusion/exclusion criteria? This is a perfect example of the role of researchers in supporting practice. Those in practice would not have the time to get to the 7 relevant articles!

Activity 10-16
Apply Findings to a Specific Practice Situation

Worksheet: Apply Evidence to a Specific Situation

Sidebar 10-2 summarizes Alex. Pretend that you and your study partners are the community mental health team serving Alex. Considering the findings of the Spencer et al. (2018) article, what will your plans be to support Alex in attending college? Complete the worksheet with your team.

Sidebar 10-2
Case Study: Alex

Alex is 14 years old. Just recently, he and his health care provider have found a stabilizing medication and therapy routine. This provides the opportunity for Alex to pursue his goal of attending college. He is also part of a mental health community that provides social and other supports.

Activity 10-17
How Might People Respond to Findings?

Worksheet: Reactions to New Data

Complete the worksheet so you are prepared for the various responses to the Spencer et al. (2018) summary article. Compare your statements with your study partners and refine your own statements based on their feedback.

Activity 10-18
Develop Take-Home Messages

Worksheet: Create Take-Home Messages

The final step in the analysis process for evidence-based practice is to summarize the findings for those who need to use the ideas to improve their practices. Professionals want clear, easy-to-understand guidelines about what to do. We will call these summaries "Take-Home Messages" to remind ourselves to use understandable language. Pretend that the articles you read were the **definitive** articles on the topic. Use the worksheet to summarize your work.

Activity 10-19
Use Legitimate Websites

Visit one of the websites (such as the Cochrane Collaboration) and scan the topics available from this website. Obtain a review to share with your study partners.

Go to one other website that provides summaries of research for professionals and consumers. Be sure that you find legitimate websites that would meet professional standards.

SUMMARY

Scholars who prepare summary and meta-analysis articles provide a great service to professionals in practice. These materials integrate findings across a large group of studies, enabling those in practice to obtain a wealth of information in one source.

Examining Evidence Related to Emerging and Controversial Practices

Another issue you will encounter in evidence-based practice is how to handle emerging and controversial practices. In this unit, you will explore this issue and learn how to obtain information and then evaluate whether a particular practice is worthy of attention as an evidence-based practice. There are two primary reasons why professionals need to understand how to examine emerging and controversial practices. First, younger disciplines like occupational therapy have not had the time to develop substantial and longitudinal evidence about their practices; data are only available about some of the profession's practices. Second, disciplines are always evolving, so new ideas are always emerging and they need to be tested. There will never be a time when we know all there is to know and have the final evidence on the effectiveness of practices.

When you complete the work for this unit, you will have the following skills and competencies:

- Learning the factors that might make a practice controversial
- Analyzing an emerging practice area to determine whether it is controversial
- Constructing a summary for colleagues to inform them about an emerging or controversial practice
- Preparing materials for families and clients to inform them about an emerging or controversial practice

You will be reviewing articles and web materials, creating summaries for comparison and contrast, gaining insights from your study partners, and creating Take-Home Messages for constituent groups.

Dunn, W., & Proffitt, R. *Bringing Evidence Into Everyday Practice: Practical Strategies for Health Care Professionals, Second Edition* (pp. 89-94).

Activity 11-1
Read the Literature

Read the articles listed here. They provide background for your work in this unit and will shed some light on how to decide about the viability of a practice.

McWilliam, R. A. (1999). Controversial practices: The need for a reacculturation of early intervention fields. Topics in Early Childhood Special Education, 19(3), 177-188. https://doi.org/10.1177%2F027112149901900310

Nickel, R. E. (1996). Controversial therapies for young children with developmental disabilities. Infants and Young Children, 8(4), 29-40. https://doi.org/10.1097/00001163-199604000-00005

Professionals know that they need to provide evidence-based practice, and you have been learning some strategies in this book. However, when new ideas emerge it is hard to know what to do with them. Has there been enough time to test the ideas? Are the new ideas based on sound foundational knowledge? How would others judge the ideas? In this unit, we will explore some ways to organize your thinking about emerging and sometimes controversial practices.

There are always new ideas forming and being tested in every profession; this is a necessary part of the evolution of a discipline and a body of knowledge. New ideas are enticing and exciting and challenge the status quo. But just because something is new doesn't mean that the ideas are preferable to current trends. When professionals have some systematic ways of considering the feasibility of new ideas for providing directions for evidence-based practice, then professionals are not subject to bias because "new" is interesting and "better."

The two readings in this unit are from interdisciplinary childhood journals. The authors provide a structure for considering whether a set of ideas will meet professional standards. These are not the only ways to analyze emerging practices; if you have others you know about, add them to your resources.

SUMMARIZING THE KEY POINTS OF THESE ARTICLES

Since these are not research articles, they do not contain the typical sections we have come to expect in an article. Instead, these authors provide a set of guidelines about how to analyze an emerging practice to decide if it is controversial.

Activity 11-2
Create a Summary

Worksheet: Summarize the Characteristics of a Research Article

Create a summary for yourself that contains brief definitions of the key points from these articles. This will serve as a tip sheet when you are analyzing a controversial or emerging practice of your own.

Activity 11-3
Handle Anomalous Data

Worksheet: Reactions to New Data

You will encounter many lively debates over emerging and controversial practices during your career. Those that are passionately in favor (or against) an emerging practice will have many things to say about their point of view. Challenging one's beliefs will be a regular part of your professional life. Some of the controversial practices cited in the McWilliam (1999) and Nickel (1996) articles may be practices you have seen implemented. Perhaps there is an emerging practice you are drawn to and want to try. Take time to think about all points of view before making any specific decisions about what you believe and how you will practice.

Select one of the controversial practices summarized in the McWilliam (1999) or Nickel (1996) articles. Refer to your Executive Summary (see Sidebar 2-1) of the Chinn and Brewer (1993) article to decide where a colleague's reactions might fall related to handling anomalous data. Bring these issues up with your study partners.

Activity 11-4
Analyze an Emerging or Controversial Practice

Worksheet: Analyze Intervention Practices to Determine Whether They Are Controversial

Now that you have some ideas about what to look for as a controversial practice, let's practice applying these ideas to a specific situation. Let's go through the steps using a particular practice. There is a practice being implemented in some occupational therapy outpatient clinics called "neurofeedback" or "brain training" for children with ADHD.

First, let's conduct an internet search (e.g., Google) on your topic. We can use search terms such as "neurofeedback," "ADHD," and "occupational therapy." Several of the hits we see are links to individual clinics and practices across the country. Some of the hits link us to scholarly articles as well as the National Center for Complementary and Integrative Health (part of the National Institutes of Health).

Now we'll explore the scholarly literature. Use a database such as CINAHL, ERIC, PsychInfo, PubMed, or Ovid. You can use the same key words, key authors, or other distinct terms used in the practice you are examining. You may need to adjust your search terms. Refer to Unit 1 and your companion texts if you need a refresher on searching professional literature databases. In our search we find a few articles and a few reviews. Most of the individual studies are lower levels of evidence and have a small number of participants. The reviews are of broader topics (e.g., complementary and alternative approaches to ADHD) and the authors make a similar conclusion: there is minimal to no evidence supporting the use of neurofeedback for children with ADHD.

Sidebar 11-1 is a summary of the searches based on the McWilliam (1999) and Nickel (1996) articles.

Sidebar 11-1

Case Study: Analyze Intervention Practices to Determine Whether They Are Controversial

Using the McWilliam (1999) and Nickel (1996) articles as a guide, analyze one emerging practice to determine whether it is controversial.

Topic

Neurofeedback, or "brain training" for children with ADHD

Summary From Google Search

There are a number of websites that come up when searching this topic. Some websites are clinics or practices. One website is the National Center for Complementary and Integrative Health. There are also a number of websites that include an option to purchase equipment.

Summary From Professional Search

There are a few studies that show positive results when comparing neurofeedback to sham treatment, but those studies do not have a large number of participants. A few reviews are published and none of them include recommendations for using neurofeedback in children with ADHD.

Analysis Based on McWilliam (1999) Criteria

McWilliam (1999) Criteria	Information From Websites
Cure Claims	*Many clinic/practitioner websites include claims that ADHD is not "curable."*
Practitioner Specialization	*No specific information, though many clinics list neuropsychologists as the expert administering the treatment.*
Questionable Research	*Many websites do not list references.*
Intensity	*Large variation in dosage (minutes/session and total number of sessions).*
Legal Action	*No indication of legal action.*

Analysis Based on Nickel (1996) Criteria

Nickel (1996) Criteria	Information From Websites
Legal Action	*No indication of legal action.*
Oversimplified Theories	*There have been no published studies indicating a mechanism of action for neurofeedback.*
Effective for Many	*Many websites include claims that people of all ages have benefited.*
Dramatic Results	*There are reports of increased focus and attention, but minimal reports of functional changes.*
Case Reports vs. Studies	*Most studies are small case reports and small pilot studies.*
Treatment Objectives	*Most studies include a single study group, some are compared to a sham treatment. Outcomes measured were attention, and focus was on contrived tests often administered right after the treatment.*
Side Effects	*No side effects were reported.*

Conclusions Regarding This Intervention Practice

There is minimal evidence to support the use of neurofeedback for children with ADHD. Although there are some published studies, the level of evidence is low. More research is needed before implementing this intervention in practice. It may be appropriate to try at a single-case level in conjunction with other treatments.

Adapted from McWilliam (1999) and Nickel (1996).

Activity 11-5
Analyze an Emerging or Controversial Practice on Your Own

Worksheet: Analyze Intervention Practices to Determine Whether They Are Controversial

Now that you have practiced this, do an analysis of an emerging or controversial practice on your own or with a group. Fill out the worksheet as you work through the steps.

Identify the practice you are curious about. This may be something you have heard about from a colleague, seen in a continuing education brochure, or saw in your social media feed. Conduct an internet search of the practice. You may need to discuss what key words to use with your study partners and/or your instructor. Select three to five sites to review and take notes on what you find, with particular attention to information that will help you conduct your "controversial therapies" analysis. Write a three- to five-sentence summary of your findings.

Next, conduct a professional literature search (e.g., CINAHL, ERIC, PsychInfo, PubMed, Ovid) using the same key words, key authors, or other distinct terms used in the practice you are examining. Remember, these resources have been independently reviewed by noninterested parties. Print the hits you get from these searches as well. Review the material and write a three- to five-sentence summary of what you find.

Now compile a summary of your findings. After you collect and review the materials, complete an analysis using McWilliam (1999) and Nickel (1996) criteria. Then, construct an overall summary statement about the emerging or controversial practice. Sidebar 11-1 is a summary of the searches based on the McWilliam (1999) and Nickel (1996) articles.

Activity 11-6
Look for Patterns and Themes

Worksheet: Summarize Key Points for Analysis

Think about the similarities and differences in the two methods of searching and the two methods for analyzing the practice. McWilliam (1999) and Nickel (1996) have some overlapping criteria and some distinct criteria—discuss these with your study partners.

- What did each author draw out of the material with their particular point of view?
- What do you know because of using both articles that you would have missed with only one article as a reference?
- What are the differences between the internet search results and the professional search results?
- Did the material support or complement each other, or were the two search methods in conflict?

Seeing the differences in these two search methods is important because many families and individuals you serve will use the internet to find out about their situation. Your job as a professional is to help families and individuals evaluate that information in light of evidence-based practice standards. Without your help, the people you serve do not know how to evaluate the information on the internet—it all looks informative and impressive to an untrained eye.

- What are the benefits and risks of this access?
- How can you, as a professional, guide families and individuals so they find legitimate information for their decision making?

Now, think about the topic.

- What happened to your thinking from before and after each of the searches?
- How did your ideas change?
- Have you observed that professionals have incorporated appropriate findings into their practices?
- Are you going to do anything differently now that you have searched and analyzed this emerging or controversial practice?

Activity 11-7
Group Discussion

Meet with your study partners and discuss your findings and reactions to the emerging and controversial practices.

Activity 11-8
Develop Take-Home Messages

Worksheet: Create Take-Home Messages

When you have completed your analysis of an emerging or controversial practice, you will need to create a summary statement about that practice. Professionals want clear, easy-to-understand guidelines about what to do. We will call these summaries "Take-Home Messages" to remind ourselves to use understandable language. You will need to consider Take-Home Messages for your colleagues (within your discipline and from other disciplines), family members, other care providers, and those receiving your care.

Select two constituent groups as the focus of your attention and create some Take-Home Messages for them. Use the worksheet to summarize your work.

When addressing emerging and controversial practices, ask yourself a few different questions:

- What would you say to colleagues about using this emerging or controversial practice?
- What would you say to your team regarding the emerging or controversial practice?
- What resources from the professional and internet literature would you want to make your colleagues aware of?
- How would you counsel a family/individual about how to evaluate the emerging or controversial practice for them?

SUMMARY

There are always new ideas emerging in professional practice. We need to consider these ideas with an open and critical eye. This unit provided you with strategies for considering these emerging trends as part of an ever-evolving professional practice.

Creating Evidence Within Your Own Practice

Throughout this book, we have been exploring ways to examine the evidence available in the professional literature. All of the skills you have learned will enable you to access the literature so you can provide evidence-based practices to the people you serve in your practice. However, regardless of whether you identify evidence to support a particular practice or not, you have the responsibility to collect data within your practice to evaluate whether a practice is effective **for that particular person/family/setting**. Even proven practices may not be the right intervention for a specific situation. In this unit you will learn some basic strategies for collecting evidence within your practice to guide your decisions about whether the interventions are effective. When you are applying evidence-based practices from the literature, your data collection confirms and verifies the effectiveness of the practice within your situation. When you are extending ideas from the literature to new populations or settings, you are creating evidence about this new application. In any case, collecting data to guide your practice is another everyday way to provide evidence-based practice.

When professionals share information with each other without data, we can call this "professional folklore." This refers to information that professionals share with each other based on their experiences and ideas without a systematic structure. Professionals passing on folklore might say "It really works when you ..." An evidence-based professional says "Studies have shown ..." or "We have some evidence that ..." We might need to add "This intervention idea hasn't been tested with children this age," or "We don't have evidence for this intervention, so let's try it for 2 weeks, measure progress, and then decide if we are going to continue." As you become more skilled at collecting data in your practice, you can share your systematic findings with colleagues. Because you have collected data, you are not passing along professional folklore, you are sharing evidence. Everyday evidence builds just as research studies build, to illustrate patterns we can rely on for better decision making.

Dunn, W., & Proffitt, R. *Bringing Evidence Into Everyday Practice: Practical Strategies for Health Care Professionals, Second Edition* (pp. 95-105). © 2024 Taylor & Francis Group.

When you complete the work for this unit, you will have the following skills and competencies:
- Understanding the importance of everyday evidence in your practice
- Learning specific strategies for collecting evidence within your practice
- Recognizing how to decide when interventions are not effective and need to be changed based on your data
- Constructing a data collection and monitoring plan that extends evidence from the literature
- Practicing reporting data-based information to colleagues and families

Basic Structure for Evidence-Based Data Collection in Your Practice

When professionals take the time to collect data, it is important to make sure that these efforts will yield useful findings. If you collect information that is unreliable, then others may not agree with or believe your conclusions. Take the time to organize your efforts so you have reliable data.

Collect Information, Not Interpretations

There are two levels of information gathering; they each have an important purpose but must not be confused with each other in evidence-based practice. The first level of information gathering is factual; anyone gathering the same information will obtain the same information. For example, if you are doing a skilled observation in a classroom, a factual observation is the number of times the student leaves their desk. Anyone watching this student would be able to see whether the student left their chair (as long as you set clear operational definitions about "leaving the chair," see Unit 3 about operational definitions).

The second level of information gathering involves making a hypothesis about what the observed behavior means. An occupational therapist using a sensory processing frame of reference might say "The student needs movement input, so they leave their chair frequently to get this movement." A teacher using a behavioral frame of reference might say "The student is trying to get my attention, so they leave their chair a lot." A psychologist using a psychosocial frame of reference might say "The student is anxious and is moving around to manage their anxiety." Professionals won't agree about this level of information gathering unless they are using the same frame of reference. When planning on an interdisciplinary team, members negotiate which hypotheses seem most plausible for the student and begin their planning based on these hypotheses. The team then establishes factual ways to collect data on the desired outcomes (e.g., in this example, the student getting his seatwork completed in a timely manner) so they can measure the accuracy of their hypothesis and the effectiveness of their intervention.

Measure Something That Matters

It is tempting to measure things that are easy to measure, but this does not advance your evidence-based practice. For example, you can count how many times a person looks away from their hands while trying to crochet, but this may not be relevant to the person getting back to a satisfying experience with their hobby of crocheting. Perhaps the person didn't previously watch their hands while crocheting and looking away gives them the chance to feel other sensory inputs while crocheting. Perhaps looking at their hands reminds them that their arthritis is bad, and this reduces their optimism about getting back to crocheting. If we are working with someone to reconnect them with their hobby of crocheting, then we have to measure the **crocheting experience** somehow. Getting at the most important factors requires some planning. In this example, you would want to ask them what makes crocheting satisfying, and then find a way to document what they tell you. If they tell you they like to stack up the squares for a blanket, you can count the number of squares (and you might have them start with small squares, so they see progress quickly). If they tell you they just like to spend some time crocheting every day, then you might record the number of minutes they crochet or the number of times per day they pick up their crocheting and ask them to rate their satisfaction each day (you would hope to see a relationship between the amount of time and increasing satisfaction to indicate you were making progress).

Measure Participation, Not Interventions

Since professionals spend a lot of time working out creative interventions, it is easy to slip into the pattern of measuring the procedures rather than the outcomes you desire. For example, if you are running a community reintegration program, you could get focused on member attendance and involvement with the training activities. This is good information for your records about the intervention and it will help you know whether those that were more involved had better outcomes—but it does not indicate effectiveness. You have to measure the desired outcomes to know the effectiveness of your intervention. In this example you might record how long it takes members to get housing or employment, and how many secure housing or employment.

Measure During Living, Not During Therapy

When we stay focused on the person's participation, it is clear that in order to know whether our interventions are effective, they must change the person's life. Changing how they performs in a clinical situation is a step toward increased competence, but it does not substitute for actual changes in participation during the times when the person really needs to participate. If we train adolescents in social skills in a planned social group, it is a good place to learn and practice (this is part of the intervention). If we want to know whether those adolescents manage better with their peers, we will have to watch them during class, in transitions between classes, in a club, or at a party. In this example, we can also rely on the adolescents to report their satisfaction with socializing because they are in the classes, hallways, clubs, and parties. You have read studies that use parent, self, or partner reports of participation in natural contexts. You can also have people videotape in the natural setting, and you can code the behaviors of interest later.

Record What You Are Measuring

Writing down what happens creates a record of your hypotheses and outcomes. When your interventions are working to improve participation, your documentation verifies this. When your interventions are not having the desired effect, documentation helps you remember your clinical reasoning processes so you can reformulate your hypotheses and plans. Find simple ways to document:

- Use bullet point lists to characterize the behaviors of interest.
- Make graphs showing the data points and progress.
- Design simple illustrations or take pictures of desired behaviors.
- Add notations to your graphs and lists so you don't have to go back to a full report or record each time you need to review your documentation.

Simple recording plans become a great communication tool for you. Everyone involved (including persons, families, and other professionals) gets the picture about what is going on very quickly.

DATA COLLECTION METHODS

Many authors have written about ways to document the effectiveness of your interventions. Let's examine a few examples and then you can practice.

Copy Measurement Strategies in Journal Articles

The first resources you have are all the intervention studies you have read or will read. When a study tests an intervention that is applicable to your practice, examine the measurement strategies they have used. Are there any that you can use in your practice to document participation outcomes? Did they make an interesting table or graph?

Activity 12-1
Let's Practice

Select a journal article whose findings are applicable to an area of practice that is interesting to you. Make a worksheet showing how you could use their measurement strategies within a practice situation.

Find Out Exactly What the Outcome Needs to Be

A big barrier to documenting the effectiveness of practices is having unclear ideas about what the desired outcome is. Families and individuals might say "We want her to walk." Does this mean getting around with a cane, using a walker, or only walking independently of other supports? When professionals don't get specific, they can be at crossed purposes to the people being served.

So, how do we get specific? We ask the right questions and listen to the answers. Here are some questions that can get you started:

- What will it look like when your parent can walk again?
- How will we know that your child has more friends?
- What would a perfect morning routine be for your family?
- What would a successful job be for you?

You will be surprised about the answers. As professionals we are predisposed to thinking about problems a certain way. Although this is mostly helpful, sometimes this characteristic can cause us to jump to incorrect conclusions. The family may think independence upon returning home means your parent can indicate what they want for dinner, while the occupational therapist may think independence means your parent has to make dinner. Intervention plans would not look the same in these two scenarios.

Activity 12-2
Let's Practice

Meet with a study partner and interview each other in this way. Start with a general statement ("I want to be more fit"). Jot notes about what you think this means, and then ask the other person what it means to them (e.g., what would "being more fit" look like for you?). Compare your answers.

Use a Reference Person to Get Ideas

Sometimes you will struggle to identify an appropriate level of a behavior for your outcome goal. In these cases, you can observe an average person in the same setting to get an idea about what would be an appropriate amount of the behavior. Let's say the family says they want their parent to socialize more. Their parent is in a nursing home; how much social interaction is appropriate during certain times of the day at the nursing home? You can go into the dining room or game room and record what other people do. What does their interaction look like (e.g., are they talking, watching, moving, smiling)? What is the frequency of these behaviors? Knowing this baseline information in concert with the parent and the family's ideas about interacting will help you craft a great measurement of his progress.

Develop a Progress Monitoring Plan

Clark et al. (2006) provide an excellent summary of the progress monitoring method (Table 12-1). They provide a six-point structure for designing a theoretically sound way to collect evidence for your practice. With a simple worksheet, you have cues about what to think about next, and soon you are finished writing your plan.

Table 12-1
Progress Monitoring Plan

Outline of Tasks for Progress Monitoring	Summary of Components
Behavior	Describe what the person is doing currently, with an emphasis on what participation is challenging.
Goal	Describe the participation goal.
Hypothesis for Observed Behavior	This is an IF… THEN statement. In the IF part, tell what your hypothesis is and link it to a theoretically sound idea. In the THEN part, tell your general intervention idea based on the theoretically sound hypothesis.
Intervention Plan	Describe specifically what your intervention will look like so other people can implement it.
Measurement Strategy	Describe how you will measure and who will measure the behavior.
Decision-Making Plan	State the criteria for success on the goal.

Let's look at an example. Stella is having a hard time with independent work in the classroom. Table 12-2 shows what the team documented for Stella.

Table 12-2
Sample Progress Monitoring Plan for Stella

Outline of Tasks for Progress Monitoring	Stella's Plan
Behavior	*Stella is constantly repositioning herself and fidgeting in her chair, making it difficult to complete her seatwork.*
Goal	*Stella will continue working independently for 10 minutes.*
Hypothesis for Observed Behavior	*IF Stella's distractibility is due to her need to obtain additional sensory input,* *THEN interventions that increase this input during independent work will make it possible for Stella to complete seatwork.*
Intervention Plan	*Provide Stella with a weighted vest, flexible cushion, and heavy lap pillow during seatwork.*
Measurement Strategy	*The teacher will record the number of minutes Stella continues working independently.*
Decision-Making Plan	*Within 5 weeks, Stella will work for 10 minutes in a row.*

Stella's team discussed their test results, observations, interviews with teachers, and an ecological assessment and hypothesized that Stella needed more intense sensory input to help her focus and complete her seatwork. They reviewed the literature and found some evidence for using weighted vests and flexible seating to improve work product to support their decisions.

This team didn't want to take any chances on having success! They added three interventions together to try to increase her participation. We might call this an "intervention package." They won't know if only one selection might have worked, they will only know if the intervention package works. You will also notice that the teacher did not care about accuracy of work in this plan. She just wanted Stella to keep working, she felt that accuracy and getting the work to be just the right level for Stella could come later. The teacher said "We can't know whether Stella has skills because she doesn't work long enough to show us what she can do." The teacher agreed to record the length of time Stella worked during independent work time and felt confident that she would make swift progress.

GRAPHING STELLA'S PROGRESS

Figure 12-1 is a simple graph to chart Stella's progress. We made a 5 (number of weeks) x 10 (number of minutes) graph to make it easy to record her time working. We drew a line from 0 to the endpoint (5 weeks and 10 minutes) to show how much progress she needed to make each week. Then the teacher could just color in the boxes indicating the average number of minutes each week.

	wk1	wk2	wk3	wk4	wk5
10					
9					
8					
7					
6					
5					
4					
3					
2					
1					

Figure 12-1. Stella's progress monitoring plan data sheet. (Reprinted from *Sensory Profile 2*. Copyright © 2014 by NCS Pearson Inc. Reproduced with permission. All rights reserved.)

We want Stella to work at least as many minutes as the diagonal line indicates for each week. She meets this standard during Weeks 1 and 2. During Week 3 she makes no more progress, but continues at the same level. The team intervenes immediately to adjust the plan so Stella will make more progress.

Activity 12-3
Let's Practice

As you can see from Figure 12-1, Stella made progress the first 2 weeks of the program, then she stalled in the third week. Because the team was collecting data, they knew right away that the intervention was only partially effective. Meet with your study partners and decide what to do next so that Stella continues to make progress during her independent work.

You might want to make a new hypothesis. What are some additional reasons why Stella could be inattentive (e.g., the work is too hard for her)? This hypothesis will guide the planning process.

Activity 12-4
Let's Practice Some More!

Worksheet: Progress Monitoring Plan

Saul is a 16-month-old boy who is happy and playful with his family. He is the only boy, with two sisters and grandparents close by. His parents are concerned that he is still not moving around by himself to play. When the team completed their assessments, they had several hypotheses about why Saul wasn't moving:

- Saul is weak when compared to age peers.
- Saul has poor biomechanical alignment and instability.
- Saul has low registration. (He misses sensory cues.)
- Saul has sensation avoiding. (He gets overwhelmed easily with sensory input.)

The family caters to Saul, so he doesn't have to move to play. Saul's family are very involved with their children. The team decided to make more than one progress monitoring plan, so they could discuss the options with the family and make the decision about where to begin with them.

Meet with your study partners and write three progress monitoring plans for Saul's family using the worksheet. Table 12-3 shows the one they wrote related to lack of strength, so pick three other hypotheses for your work.

Table 12-3
Sample Progress Monitoring Plan for Saul

Outline of Tasks for Progress Monitoring	Saul's Plan
Behavior	Saul doesn't move; he sits in one place to play.
Goal	Saul will move to play with toys.
Hypothesis for Observed Behavior	IF Saul's immobility is due to lack of strength, THEN improving his strength will enable him to move to play.
Intervention Plan	Provide progressively more resistance to Saul's play schemas, including use of gravity.
Measurement Strategy	Saul will reach for and obtain toys from surfaces above his head (later we will have the family move toys to other positions that require both reaching and shifting body position).
Decision-Making Plan	Within a month, Saul will obtain a toy from a surface above shoulder level within 10 seconds of a cue.

Adapted from *Sensory Profile 2.* Copyright © 2014 by NCS Pearson Inc.

DESIGN A CHART OR GRAPH TO RECORD BEHAVIOR

The progress monitoring plans typically invite the team to make a graph of the behavior. You can make charts for just about anything. Visual prompts about progress are helpful because they serve as a reminder about the goal and show what progress we are making.

Activity 12-5
Let's Practice

Chart your own progress on something: make a chart showing which food groups you have had in your diet each day, or graph the times you remember where your keys are. How do graphing and charting change your behavior?

When you go into a practice situation, create a way to graph the progress of a person you are serving. Share the graph with the individual and see how that changes the behavior.

DEVELOP A SPECIFIC SCALE FOR OUTCOME ATTAINMENT

Some research programs use a method called goal-attainment scaling. When using this method in research, there are very specific criteria about how to establish the scale. The precision is related to making sure that each step along the scale represents exactly the same amount of change as every other step along the scale.

We can take this idea and adapt it for the purpose of documenting progress.

- First you identify the current behavior. This behavior becomes the -1 point on the scale.
- Then you ask "How would the behavior look if it got worse?" This behavior becomes -2 on the scale.
- Next, you ask "What will the behavior look like when we have reached our goal?". This becomes the neutral (or 0) point on the scale.
- Next, find out what a dream behavioral outcome would be. "What would the behavior look like if we exceeded our expectations?". This becomes the +1 point on the scale.
- If you like, you can go to utopia and ask one more question "If this person had perfect behavior, what would it look like?". This is the +2 point on the scale.

Now you have a ready-made way to document progress on behaviors that might be too complicated to characterize other ways.

Let's look at an example. Kim has trouble with the bus. She is disruptive with her classmates when they are going to the bus at the end of the school day. Figure 12-2 is an example of what the teacher, parent, bus driver, and principal came up with for their outcome scale.

-2	-1	0	+1	+2
Worse	**Current**	**Goal**	**Exceeds Goal**	**Utopia!**
Kim has to be pulled out of the bus line and have her parents pick her up.	*Kim pushes and bumps people while going to the bus.*	*Kim gets to the bus without incident.*	*Kim gets to the bus and is seated without incident.*	*Kim gets positive reports about the bus ride after getting on the bus without incident.*

Figure 12-2. Example of how a Goal Attainment Scale would be operationalized.

The team laughed about the utopia possibility and thought it was silly to write it down. But an interesting thing happened: by talking about the specific behaviors (they had a list of what "without incident" meant and a list of "positive bus behaviors") among themselves and with Kim, she started to remind everyone when she did one of the behaviors (e.g., "I said something nice to the driver today"). So, consider the long view when you do this yourself.

The principal and bus driver made the judgments each day, and the teacher made a chart with Kim showing her progress. They did it on a computer program so they could email it to Kim's parents as well, providing an additional way to reinforce desirable behaviors.

This outcome attainment plan does not tell us what interventions the team used to change Kim's behavior; it focuses attention on measuring the participation, and that is what will indicate how effective the interventions were.

Activity 12-6
Let's Practice

Think of something you want to improve about yourself or your life. Write an outcome attainment scale for this area of your life. Post it in a prominent place, so you remember what you want to accomplish. Use graph paper to graph your progress.

RECORD OUTCOMES IN CONTEXT

An ecological assessment is an evaluation of the contexts in which behaviors occur. As professionals, we want to look for situations that are easier and harder for the persons we are serving, so we can tailor our recommendations accordingly. We think about what might be contributing to or interfering with participation in each setting of interest.

When designing data collection to document the effectiveness of our interventions, contexts matter as well. Here is an example of an ecological assessment for a young woman who wants to make more friends. Assessments indicated that she is sensitive to noise in her environment. The therapist wants to identify settings that were more or less likely to support making new friends.

Figure 12-3 is a shortened version of an ecological assessment. The therapist and the woman decide that lunch and after work have the biggest potential for developing friends, and that the woman has some control over these situations. The intervention is the therapist making recommendations to the woman about how to manage her auditory sensitivity to maximize the possibility of being able to interact successfully. The measurement of outcomes in this example will be related to the woman's satisfaction with developing friends (e.g., number of times per week she goes out to lunch with others, number of people she visits with after work).

	Riding the Bus to Work	Working at the Office	Going to Lunch	Socializing After Work
Auditory Sensitivity	*Lots of people talking, moving around, bus noises as people enter and exit*	*Has own office with a door* *Plays soft music in the background*	*Variable, depending on where she eats* *Invitation to join big groups may trigger sensitivity*	*Venues vary and therefore have varying levels of sound*

Figure 12-3. Example of an ecological assessment for auditory sensitivity across the workday.

RECORD PERFORMANCE AND SATISFACTION WITH PERFORMANCE

The Canadian Occupational Performance Measure (COPM; Law et al., 1990) evaluates a person's level of performance and the person's satisfaction with current performance. There are data on the COPM itself, documenting its ability to record changes in participation. Combining performance with satisfaction is a way to acknowledge that people can be satisfied with average performance in some aspects of their lives. The COPM is a great tool for documenting the effectiveness of an intervention in daily life.

SUMMARY

In this unit, you learned some basic ways to collect data within your practice so you can document the actual progress being made. Collecting data is a way to verify the effectiveness of your evidence-based practice decisions and extends the literature into the lives of the people you are serving.

Communicating Evidence
Critical Conversations

You have created Take-Home Messages as an activity in multiple units and you probably now feel comfortable distilling the most important points from an article or a group of articles. Being able to summarize evidence related to clinical practice is an important and necessary skill. As you encounter evidence in practice and other courses as a student, you may find yourself summarizing the main points of the article without prompting. You are also becoming more aware of your own reactions to anomalous data. You may also observe how other health care professionals react to the same evidence or data, noting that their reaction may be different from yours. All of these skills are important to evidence-based practice.

As you learned in Unit 1 and from the readings in Law and MacDermid (2014), evidence-based practice is a triad of evidence, clinical experience, and client values and preferences. This textbook has focused mainly on the "evidence" component of the triad. We would be remiss if we did not address *how* to integrate all we have learned about evidence with your clinical expertise and the values of your clients.

During this unit, you will practice communicating your Take-Home Messages to a variety of people including clients, their trusted support person, and other health care professionals. You will work through more difficult conversations with other health care professionals, including those in occupational therapy who may be more reluctant to using evidence in practice.

When you complete the work for this unit, you will have the following skills and competencies:
- Communicating Take-Home Messages for a variety of stakeholder groups
- Hypothesizing how others might respond to anomalous data and construct appropriate responses
- Critiquing the performance of your peers in sharing Take-Home Messages and adjust your own performance accordingly
- Understanding how communicating evidence fits into the evidence-based practice triad

Dunn, W., & Proffitt, R. *Bringing Evidence Into Everyday Practice: Practical Strategies for Health Care Professionals, Second Edition* (pp. 107-112). © 2024 Taylor & Francis Group.

You will be revising Take-Home Messages, practicing giving Take-Home Messages to various groups, critiquing performance of peers, considering reactions to anomalous data, and creating scripts for Take-Home Messages related to areas of minimal evidence.

Activity 13-1
Review a Take-Home Message

Select a Take-Home Message worksheet from a prior activity in this textbook. Locate the article(s) used to create the Take-Home Message worksheet. Re-read the article(s) to familiarize yourself with the topic.

Activity 13-2
Compare and Contrast

Worksheet: Compare and Contrast Take-Home Messages

Complete the first column of the worksheet using the article from the worksheet. If you can't find the information in the article, use your best guess, or follow the directions here to help describe the study population demographics.

Evidence Detective Tip

Most articles use Table 1 to describe the demographics of the study population. The study inclusion and exclusion criteria can provide additional details as to who took part in the study.

Now, think about a population to whom the findings of the study might apply. This may be a client population that you work with regularly. If you are not in practice yet, think about the population where you work or live. Fill in the second column of the Compare and Contrast Take-Home Messages worksheet based on that population. You can use online websites to help discover demographic information you don't know.

LOOKING FOR PATTERNS AND THEMES

First, look for similarities and differences between the article's participants and your client population.
- How do the populations compare? What are the similarities?
- How do the populations diverge? How different are they? Is it a large or small difference?

The answers to these questions can help you understand how to use the findings. For example, the article might have focused on a rural population and you work in a large, urban city. What does this mean when you think about the approach the researchers took to recruit study participants?

What about specific methods for delivering the intervention? How much of a role do you think demographic variables such as race/ethnicity and age played in interpreting the study findings? You can use your answers to these questions to begin formulating hypotheses for your practice. Complete the third column of the worksheet as you compare and contrast the article's participants and your client population.

Now, think about your Take-Home Message worksheet.

- What happened to your thinking from before and after completing the worksheet?
- How did your ideas change?
- How might you adjust your Take-Home Messages to better match your client population?

Be prepared to discuss your ideas and thoughts with your study partners. Practice saying your new Take-Home Messages with your study partners.

Now, consider what your client population might have to say about your Take-Home Messages.

Activity 13-3
Adapt Take-Home Messages

Worksheet: Create Take-Home Messages

First, conduct an internet search (e.g., Google) on your topic. Save the hits you get from each search. You may need to discuss what key words to use with your study partners and/or your instructor. Select three to five sites to review and take notes on what you find. Write a three- to five-sentence summary of your findings.

Think about the summary of your internet search. What questions do you think your clients and/or their trusted supports/caregivers might have if they were do a similar internet search? Think back to the responses to anomalous data from prior units. How can you adjust your Take-Home Messages to address potential questions from your client population? Write a summary of the changes you made.

Activity 13-4
Practice With Your Study Partners

By now you have adjusted your Take-Home Messages a few times to better reflect the clients you serve (or will someday serve). Pretend your study partners are your client and/or their trusted support/caregiver. Practice saying your new Take-Home Messages. How did you do? How long did it take you? What part was the hardest? Ask your study partners to give you feedback and practice again. Try to get your message down to less than 2 minutes.

Swap roles. Now that you are the client and/or their trusted support/caregiver, think about questions and feelings you have. Give your study partners feedback on their delivery of the Take-Home Messages.

After you are happy with your scripts, share them with the rest of the class so you each have several examples of different approaches to get the same critical information across quickly. You can use these samples to craft messages on fieldwork and in your jobs.

As a group, reflect on the process. What were similarities and differences in approaches across students? Which samples were the most influential to your thinking? How can you use these examples in the future?

Activity 13-5
Review a Take-Home Message

Worksheet: Reactions to New Data

Select a new Take-Home Message worksheet from a prior unit's activity in this textbook.
Locate the article(s) used to create the Take-Home Message worksheet.
Re-read the article(s) to familiarize yourself with the topic.

Activity 13-6
Adapt Take-Home Messages

Consider your Take-Home Messages. How do you see occupational therapy being represented in your messages? Are there specific measures or intervention strategies that are highly specific to occupational therapy? What role did an occupational therapist play in the intervention within those studies? If the intervention was not conducted by an occupational therapist, how do you think it could be adapted by an occupational therapist? What value does occupational therapy bring to the client population/practice setting in the study? These questions will be easier or harder to answer depending on the article you chose. Studies that are published outside of occupational therapy literature may require more thought and discussion. Write a three- to five-sentence summary of the distinct value of occupational therapy in your article.

Imagine that you are part of an interdisciplinary team that works with the client population in the article. You are the only occupational therapist on the team and you want to talk with the team about the article in your Create Take-Home Messages worksheet. Think about your summary of the distinct value of occupational therapy. How can you adjust your Take-Home Messages to ensure that the team understands the unique and distinct value of occupational therapy? Write a summary of the changes you made.

Activity 13-7
Practice With Your Study Partners

Worksheet: Create Take-Home Messages

Pretend your study partners are team members from a different discipline. Practice saying your new Take-Home Messages. How did you do? How long did it take you? What part was the hardest? Ask your study partners to give you feedback, and practice again.

Swap roles. Now that you are an interdisciplinary team member, think about questions and feelings you have. How did your study partner do in describing the distinct role and value of occupational therapy? Give your study partners feedback on their delivery of the Take-Home Messages. As a group, reflect on the process.

Activity 13-8
Thinking About Reactions From Others

Worksheet: Your Response to Others' Reactions to New Data

Up until now we have considered how to adjust Take-Home Messages for clients, caregivers, and other team members who are from other disciplines. Unfortunately, much of the biggest "push-backs" that occupational therapists (particularly new graduates) receive when trying to implement new ideas and interventions in practice is from other occupational therapists. As we explored in earlier units, new information can be threatening and scary, especially when it directly conflicts with ideas we value.

In earlier units we considered what our own reactions are to anomalous data. Now let's consider how others in occupational therapy might react to new information we present to them.

Refer to your Executive Summary (see Sidebar 2-1) of the Chinn and Brewer (1993) article to decide where the reactions to the article from occupational therapy colleagues might occur. Complete the worksheet with those reactions. Note that there is a new column in the worksheet that is different from prior units. In the new column, think about how you would respond to an occupational therapy colleague. For example, if your colleague is likely to hold the data in abeyance, your response to that could be to set up a follow-up meeting to discuss the article/intervention after they have some time to reflect on the new information. Be prepared to discuss the ideas you have with your study partners.

Activity 13-9
Respond to Reactions From Others

Worksheet: Your Response to Others' Reactions to New Data

Some of the reactions from your occupational therapy colleagues may require thoughtful responses from you. For example, how do you respond to a colleague who flat-out rejects your suggestions for implementing a new intervention in practice, stating "This is the way we've always done it." Conversations around new evidence can be difficult, especially for new graduates.

When we consider the evidence-based practice triad (see Law & MacDermid, 2014, Chapter 1), a new graduate has skills in reading and appraising evidence for practice but has minimal clinical experience. An occupational therapy practitioner who has been in practice for 25 years has a vast amount of clinical experience, understands the needs of their clients, but may not be as current in searching for and appraising evidence for clinical practice. Let's take some time to practice having these important conversations while considering the interplay of all three components of evidence-based practice.

Activity 13-10
Practice With Your Study Partners

Pretend your study partners are occupational therapy colleagues who are skeptical of your Take-Home Messages and the intervention you want to try in practice. Create a flexible script that you can modify for different interventions and practice settings. You can find a template in Sidebar 13-1 to help you craft your script. Be sure to touch on all components of the evidence-based practice triad.

For example, part of your script might include a recognition of the many years of experience your colleague has. Maybe you can ask them about the challenges they faced when they were starting out in practice. Practice your script with your study partners or with your class and instruction. How did you do? Which part was the hardest? Ask your study partners to give you feedback and practice again. As a group, reflect on the process.

Sidebar 13-1
Template for Flexible Script of Conversations With Occupational Therapy Colleagues

- Thank them for their time.
- Set the goal of the meeting (e.g., "I want to talk about a new intervention").
- State how your colleague has contributed to the field and your practice.
- Describe intervention and study findings (the Take-Home Messages).
- Link back to how the intervention fits with the needs of your client.
- Ask them for their thoughts and opinions.

SUMMARY

In this unit, you learned about revising Take-Home Messages for various stakeholders including the clients you serve (or will serve), other health care professionals, and colleagues in the occupational therapy profession. You practiced delivering those Take-Home Messages and created scripts for difficult conversations. These conversations are part of the critical step of implementing research evidence into practice. Save these scripts to use on fieldwork and in your first job. Making adjustments to a drafted script is sometimes easier than starting over each time.

Appendix

Dunn, W., & Proffitt, R. *Bringing Evidence Into Everyday Practice: Practical Strategies for Health Care Professionals, Second Edition* (pp. 113-148). © 2024 Taylor & Francis Group.

MASTER LIST OF WORKSHEETS BY UNIT

Analyze and Improve the Precision of Participant Criteria . . . . .Unit 3

Analyze Intervention Practices to Determine Whether They Are Controversial . . . Unit 11

Analyze the Results Section of an Article . . . . .Unit 9

Apply Evidence to a Specific Situation . . . . Unit 10

Compare and Contrast Take-Home Messages . . . . Unit 13

Compare Evidence Classification Systems . . . . .Unit 1

Compare Intervention Programs . . . . .Unit 8

Create a Rationale for Summary Points From an Article. . . . . .Unit 7

Create Take-Home Messages. . . . . Units 3, 4, 5, 6, 7, 8, 9, 10, 11, and 13

Examine the Similarities and Differences in the Summary Tables . . . . .Unit 3

Examine Ways to Expand Knowledge About Assistive Devices. . . . . .Unit 4

Find Similarities in Conceptual Themes . . . . .Unit 6

Find Unique Themes Across Studies . . . . .Unit 6

Identify Answerable and Unanswerable Questions . . . . Units 3, 4, 5, 6, 7, 8, and 9

Identify Familiar Research Concepts . . . . .Unit 1

Identify New Research Concepts . . . . .Unit 1

Identify Search Parameters in a Summary Study . . . . Unit 10

Integrate Data About Smart Devices From a Systematic Review . . . . .Unit 4

List Evidence-Based Practice Concepts . . . . .Unit 1

List Steps in Implementing Evidence-Based Practice . . . . .Unit 1

Look for Themes Across Studies: Part 1 . . . . .Unit 5

Look for Themes Across Studies: Part 2 . . . . .Unit 5

Progress Monitoring Plan . . . . Unit 12

Reactions to New Data . . . . .Units 2, 3, 4, 5, 6, 7, 8, 9, 10, 11, and 13

Review the Parts of a Research Article . . . . .Unit 3

Summarize Intervention Studies. . . . . .Unit 3

Summarize Key Points for Analysis. . . . . Unit 11

Summarize the Characteristics of a Research Article. . . . . . Units 3, 4, 5, 6, 7, 8, 9, and 11

Summarize the Inclusion Criteria . . . . .Unit 3

Summarize Themes in the Introduction . . . . .Unit 3

Summary Table for Sensory Processing Patterns . . . . .Unit 7

Write Brief Take-Home Messages . . . . .Unit 3

Your Response to Others' Reactions to New Data. . . . . .Units 2 and 13

Worksheet	Unit												
	1	2	3	4	5	6	7	8	9	10	11	12	13
Analyze and Improve			X										
Analyze Intervention											X		
Analyze the Results									X				
Apply Evidence										X			
Compare and Contrast													X
Compare Evidence	X												
Compare Intervention								X					
Create a Rationale							X						
Create Take-Home Messages			X	X	X	X	X	X	X	X	X		X
Examine the Similarities			X										
Examine Ways				X									
Find Similarities						X							
Find Unique Themes						X							
Identify Answerable			X	X	X	X	X	X	X				
Identify Familiar	X												
Identify New	X												
Identify Search										X			
Integrate Data				X									
List Evidence-Based	X												
List Steps	X												
Look for Themes 1					X								
Look for Themes 2					X								
Progress Monitoring Plan												X	
Reactions to New Data		X	X	X	X	X	X	X	X	X	X		X
Review the Parts			X										
Summarize Intervention			X										
Summarize Key Points											X		
Summarize the Characteristics			X	X	X	X	X	X	X		X		
Summarize the Inclusion			X										
Summarize Themes			X										
Summary Table							X						
Write Brief			X										
Your Response		X											X

Analyze and Improve the Precision of Participant Criteria

Inclusion Criteria*	What Questions Do You Have About the Criteria? How Do You Think the Authors Would Verify That Someone Had Met This Inclusion Criteria?	How Would You Make the Criteria More Precise and Observable/ Verifiable?
Ages 18 to 55 years		
More than 6 months since TBI		
Displayed depressive symptoms (based on physician report)		
Able to communicate and follow verbal instructions in English		
No active substance abuse, psychiatric diagnosis, or suicidal ideation		
No medical conditions that would contraindicate participation		
No musculoskeletal or cognitive impairments that would limit participation		

*Data source: Schwandt, M., Harris, J. E., Thomas, S., Keightley, M., Snaiderman, A., & Colantonio, A. (2012). Feasibility and effect of aerobic exercise for lowering depressive symptoms among individuals with traumatic brain injury: A pilot study. *Journal of Head Trauma Rehabilitation, 27*(2), 99-103. https://doi.org/10.1097/HTR.0b013e31820e6858

Analyze Intervention Practices to Determine Whether They Are Controversial

Using the McWilliam (1999) and Nickel (1996) articles as a guide, analyze one emerging practice to determine whether it is controversial.

Topic:

Summary From Google Search:

Summary From Professional Search:

Analysis Based on McWilliam (1999) Criteria:

McWilliam (1999) Criteria	Information From Websites
Cure Claims	
Practitioner Specialization	
Questionable Research	
Intensity	
Legal Action	

Analysis Based on Nickel (1996) Criteria:

Nickel (1996) Criteria	Information From Websites
Legal Action	
Oversimplified Theories	
Effective for Many Dramatic Results	
Case Reports vs. Studies	
Treatment Objectives	
Side Effects	

Conclusions Regarding This Intervention Practice:

Adapted from McWilliam (1999) and Nickel (1996).

Analyze the Results Section of an Article

Exact Words From the Article Describing the Results	Explanation of Results From Filipova et al. (2015)
Sphericity assumption, tested by means of Mauchly's test, was violated consequently, Greenhouse-Geisser correction was applied in the evaluation of within-subjects factors.	
The interaction of "time" and "therapy" factors was not statistically significant for the variables DASH and flexion.	
...which could be attributed to a considerable discrepancy of initial values between both groups and an almost full mobility of the wrist attained after the therapy in both groups.	

Apply Evidence to a Specific Situation

Discuss with your study partners what you will plan for the person's program based on their particular situation and the findings in the summary article you are studying right now. Provide a rationale for your decisions. Write a script of what you will say to the person as you discuss the plan. (This is another form of Take-Home Messages!)

Decision	Rationale	What Will You Say to Them?

Compare and Contrast Take-Home Messages

Demographic Variable	Take-Home Message Article	Your Selected Client Population	Compare and Contrast
Average Age	Participants from Velligan et al. (2006) were aged 18 to 60 years old.	I see clients aged 16 to 90 years old. My oldest client is 76.	The study participants and my clients are adults, but the study participants are younger than my clients. Some of the intervention strategies might need to be adapted for my older clients.
Race and Ethnicity			
Socioeconomic Status			
Other Population Variables (Rural vs. Urban, Language Spoken)			
Diagnosis/Conditions (Including Subtypes, Years Since Incidence/ Diagnosis, Acute vs. Chronic)			
Treatment Setting			
Role of Occupational Therapist			
Social Support for Client (Type, Availability)			

Compare Evidence Classification Systems

Compare and contrast the three evidence classification systems from Activity 1-9.

	Centre for Evidence-Based Medicine (OCEBM Levels of Evidence Working Group)	Research Pyramid (Tomlin & Borgetto, 2011)	GRADE Guidelines (Balshem et al., 2011)
Briefly describe the classification system.			
What is the highest level of evidence in the system? The lowest?			
Does the system account for different types of research questions? If so, how?			
How does the system consider qualitative research?			
How easy is it for you to understand the differences in levels of evidence?			
How much does the system relate to your occupational therapy practice?			

Compare Intervention Programs

Feature	Kitago et al. (2013)	Klingels et al. (2013)	Your Article
Length of time spent with restraint	*2 wks CIMT at home under physical therapist supervision (4 hrs/day x 10 days)*	*50 hours of constraint with a splint, 1 hr at a time/ 5 times a wk, 10 wks duration*	
Length of intervention period			
Type of restraint			

Summary Statement About Constraint-Induced Therapy Procedures:

Create a Rationale for Summary Points From an Article

Here are the key points from the Little et al. (2016) article. First, restate these points in everyday words, something you could tell your neighbor, your grandparent who worked in another field, etc.

Now develop a rationale, with references, for these conclusions. Share with your study partners, and refine your lists.

Key Messages From Little et al. (2016)	How Would You Say This to Your Grandparent?	What Is Your Rationale (With References) for the Authors Making These Statements?
Five sensory subtypes emerged in the general population of children		
Subtypes differed by intensity and distribution of sensory features		
All subtypes included children with and without conditions		
Most subtypes are similar to those identified in ASD-only studies		
Subtypes may reflect the variability in all children, not just those with conditions		

Create Take-Home Messages

Pretend that the articles you just read are the definitive articles about the topic. Develop Take-Home Messages showing what you would say to a particular constituent group regarding the topic based on the articles you have read.

Take-Home Messages About	
Name: These messages are for: _____ adults receiving care _____ care providers _____ children receiving care _____ family members	
Take-Home Message	**Rationale for This Message From the Literature**

Examine the Similarities and Differences in the Summary Tables

Comparing the entries for:

	From Liu et al. (2013)	From Berger et al. (2013)	My Comments
Level/design/ participants			
Study objectives			
Intervention and outcome measures			
Results			
Study limitations			

Adapted from Liu et al. (2013) and Berger et al. (2013).

Examine Ways to Expand Knowledge About Assistive Devices

Finding From an Intervention Study About Assistive Devices (Campbell & Nolfi, 2005 and Gellis et al., 2012)	Expansion of Findings Using Bickmore et al. (2005)	Expansion of Findings Using Demeris et al. (2004)	Expansion of Findings Using Reeder et al. (2013)
Participants who received the telehealth intervention had a positive reception because they knew they could access their health care provider at any time via telehealth.	*The relationship between provider and client is important to outcomes regardless of medium (technology vs. not).*	*Include additional training on telehealth and related devices when using with the older adult population.*	*There may be additional considerations, such as perceived need and usability that may impact technology adoption.*

Find Similarities in Conceptual Themes

Concept/ Theme and Rationale for Decision	Study 1	Study 2	Study 3

Find Unique Themes Across Studies

In the boxes, enter the unique concepts to one study and your hypothesis about why this happened.

Study 1	Study 2	Study 3

Identify Answerable and Unanswerable Questions

Identify two answerable and two unanswerable questions from the Peiris et al. (2013) article. Discuss your ideas with your study partners. One example is provided.

Answerable Questions From These Articles	
Answerable Question	**What in the Article Enables You to Answer This Question?**
Does the addition of Saturday rehab visits change outcomes?	*They measured functional independence, and the Monday to Saturday group had higher scores at the end of the study.*

Unanswerable Questions From These Articles	
Unanswerable Question	**What Else Would We Need to Be Able to Answer This Question?**
How does a shorter length of stay by 2 days matter to a person and the family?	*The researchers would have to interview the participants and their families to find out whether it mattered and if so, how?*

Identify Familiar Research Concepts

List three research concepts that were already familiar to you. Then make notes about where you have encountered these concepts before.

Familiar Research Concept	Where I Have Encountered This Concept Before
Research uses objectivity to avoid bias	*High school science class experiments*
1.	
2.	
3.	

Identify New Research Concepts

List three research concepts that are new to you. Look up some additional information about this concept and make notes that will help you remember this concept in the future.

New Research Concept	What I Have Learned About This Concept
Basic research is concerned with generating ideas regardless of their application to practical problems.	*The concepts generated from basic research can be helpful in guiding ideas for applied research studies.*
1.	
2.	
3.	

Identify Search Parameters in a Summary Study

Area of Consideration	Search Criteria
Occupational Performance	
Well-Being	
Theory-Based	
Types of Studies Allowed	
Data That Must Be Present	
Participant Criteria	

Integrate Data About Smart Devices
From a Systematic Review With an Intervention Study

Barrier From Yusif et al. (2016)	Findings From Reeder et al. (2013)
Cost	Some participants commented on cost as a barrier. Some noted that $25 was too much for the device; however, others indicated that they would be willing to buy the medication dispenser.

List Evidence-Based Practice Concepts

List four ideas about evidence-based practice from the chapters. Jot down an example from practice that illustrates the concept being implemented.

Evidence-Based Practice Idea	Example of This Idea Being Implemented
Evidence-based practice is a combination of clinical expertise and evidence from the literature.	*A team of rehab therapists would discuss what to do about a patient who has had a stroke; they discuss their experiences with other patients and an article on constraint-induced therapy.*
1.	
2.	
3.	
4.	

List Steps in Implementing Evidence-Based Practice

List the five steps for implementing evidence-based practice based on the evidence-based practice forum articles you read (Activity 1-4). Then list one or two tips to remember about each step. An example is provided.

Evidence-Based Practice Steps	Tip to Remember About This Step
1. Create a clinical question.	Include: a. The occupational performance issue b. The assessment strategies c. The interventions you are wondering about (Tickle-Degnen, 1999)
2.	a. b. c.
3.	a. b. c.
4.	a. b. c.
5.	a. b. c.

Look for Themes Across Studies: Part 1

Looking for Common Concepts Across Studies

Concept That Occurs Across Studies	Where That Concept Comes From
Specifically focused training with adaptations leads to better functional and social outcomes.	*Individualized environmental supports improve functional behaviors for people with schizophrenia (Velligan et al., 2006).* *Global and social cognition improved when using compensatory cognitive strategies (Mendella et al., 2015).* *1:1 tutorials related to the technology and devices improved overall satisfaction with telehealth service (Gellis et al., 2012).* *Personalized training in using the internet for accessing health care information for older adults leads to an increased sense of control of their own health (Campbell & Nolfi, 2005).*

Look for Themes Across Studies: Part 2
Looking for Ways to Extend Knowledge
From One Area of Practice to Another

Concept From Study	That Can Be Joined With Another Study Finding	That Would Improve Intervention to Another Group
Specific training in adaptations and devices improves function and use (Velligan et al., 2006).	Older adults recognize the importance of smart home technologies in contributing to their overall health and safety, but are concerned with user-friendliness of the devices (Demeris et al., 2004).	So, we could do specific training on accessing smart home devices and how to customize available devices to meet their home environments and daily routines.

Progress Monitoring Plan

Outline of Tasks for Progress Monitoring	Plan for: Participation Focus:
Behavior	
Goal	
Hypothesis for Observed Behavior	
Intervention Plan	
Measurement Strategy	
Decision-Making Plan	

Reactions to New Data
Using Chinn and Brewer's (1993) Strategies

Think of an example from practice that would illustrate a professional using each of Chinn and Brewer's (1993) ways of responding to anomalous data.

Chinn and Brewer (1993) Responses	Examples From Practice
IGNORE the data. (Don't even bother to "explain" data away.)	
REJECT the data. (Articulate an explanation for why data should be rejected.)	
EXCLUDE the data from the domain of current beliefs. (The data are outside the domain of current beliefs.)	
Hold the data in ABEYANCE. (I promise to deal with it later. Assume that someday current beliefs will be articulated so that it can explain these data.)	
REINTERPRET the data while retaining current beliefs. (Accept the data as something that should be explained by current beliefs. Opposing forces accept data but interpret the data differently based on their own beliefs.)	
Reinterpret the data and MAKE PERIPHERAL CHANGES to current belief. (Make a relatively minor change to current belief, accepts the data but is unwilling to give up current belief and accept new beliefs.)	
Accept the data and CHANGE current beliefs, possibly in favor of a particular new belief. (Change one or more of the core aspects of current beliefs, when faced with information that is contradictory to current beliefs, accepts alternate beliefs.)	

Review the Parts of a Research Article

Parts of the Research Article	Your Reactions to the Material
Schwandt, M., Harris, J. E., Thomas, S., Keightley, M., Snaiderman, A., & Colantonio, A. (2012). Feasibility and effect of aerobic exercise for lowering depressive symptoms among individuals with traumatic brain injury: A pilot study. *Journal of Head Trauma Rehabilitation, 27*(2), 99-103. https://doi.org/10.1097/HTR.0b013e31820e6858	
Title/Abstract What do you think this article is about from reading the title and abstract only?	
Introduction Does the literature seem relevant to the topic? What convinces you that this study needs to be done to fill a gap in the literature? How have your ideas changed about what this study is about?	
Methods Could another researcher conduct this study from the information provided? What are you wondering about after reading the Methods? Now what do you think this study is about?	
Results How would you tell someone else what the findings are? What practices might you change because of these findings?	
Discussion What does the author add to the story in this section? What surprises you about the author's insights and conclusions?	

Summarize Intervention Studies

Citation	Number of Participants	Characteristics of Participants	Design Elements	Intervention Specifications	Outcome Measures	Findings

Citation: Put the reference here.
Number of Participants: Put the number of participants here.
Characteristics of Participants: List the important characteristics of participants.
Design Elements: Describe what type of comparisons or relationships are being tested/studied.
Intervention Specifications: List the most important aspects of the procedures being tested.
Outcome Measures: List the outcome measures here.
Findings: List the most important outcomes.

Adapted from Berger et al. (2013) and Liu et al. (2013).

Summarize Key Points for Analysis

Criteria From McWilliam (1999)	Definition	Examples/Notes
1.		
2.		
3.		
4.		
5.		

Criteria From Nickel (1996)	Definition	Examples/Notes
1.		
2.		
3.		
4.		
5.		

Other Notes:

Summarize the Characteristics of a Research Article

Summarize the article Finlayson, M., Preissner, K., Cho, C., & Plow, M. (2011). Randomization trial of a teleconference-delivered fatigue management program for people with multiple sclerosis. *Multiple Sclerosis Journal, 17*(9), 1130–1140. https://doi.org/10.1177/1352458511404272

Citation	Participants	Setting	Measures	Design	Intervention	Findings	Notes
Finlayson et al. (2011)							

Citation: Put the reference here.
Participants: List the important characteristics of participants.
Setting: Describe the location of the study.
Measures: List the outcome measures used in the study.
Design: Describe what type of comparisons or relationships are being tested/studied.
Intervention: List the most important aspects of the procedures being tested.
Findings: List the most important outcomes.
Notes: If you have insights or questions, jot them down.

Summarize the Inclusion Criteria

Summarize the inclusion criteria in your own words.

Summarize Themes in the Introduction

Write a phrase summarizing the theme of each paragraph in the Introduction.

1.

2.

3.

Summary Table for Sensory Processing Patterns

Article	Sample	Research Questions	No. Factors	Description of Factors
DeSantis, A., Harkins, D., Tronick, E., Kaplan, E., & Beeghly, M. (2011). Exploring an integrative model of infant behavior: What is the relationship among temperament, sensory processing, and neurobehavioral measures? *Infant Behavior and Development, 34*(2), 280-292.				
Lane, A. E., Molloy, C. A., & Bishop, S. L. (2014). Classification of children with Autism Spectrum Disorder by sensory subtype: A case for sensory-based phenotypes. *Autism Research, 7*(3), 322-333.				
Little, L. M., Dean, E., Tomchek, S. D., & Dunn, W. (2016). Classifying sensory profiles of children in the general population. *Child: Care, Health and Development, 43*(1), 81-88.				
Tomchek, S., Little, L. M., Myers, J., & Dunn, W. (2018). Sensory Subtypes in preschool aged children with autism spectrum disorder. *Journal of Autism and Developmental Disorders, 48*(6), 2139-2147.				
Uljarevic, M., Lane, A., Kelly, A., & Leekam, S. (2016). Sensory subtypes and anxiety in older children and adolescents with autism spectrum disorder. *Autism Research, 9*(10).				

Write Brief Take-Home Messages

Peiris, C. L., Shields, N., Brusco, N. K., Watts, J. J., & Taylor, N. F. (2013). Additional Saturday rehabilitation improved functional independence and quality of life and reduces length of stay. A randomized controlled trial. *BMC Medicine, 11*(1), 1-11. https://doi.org/10.1186/1741-7015-11-198

Write a three- to five-sentence summary of the findings of the article.

Write a one- to two-sentence statement for a colleague searching for an effective reaching intervention strategy.

Write a one- to two-sentence statement for a teacher who wants to try one of these strategies in their classroom.

Write a one- to two-sentence statement for a parent who heard about one of these strategies and wants you to implement the strategy with their child.

Your Response to Others' Reactions to New Data

Think about how your occupational therapy colleague might react to the article. Based on Chinn and Brewer's (1993) ways of responding to anomalous data, what would you say their reaction illustrates? What is your response to their reaction?

Chinn and Brewer (1993) Responses		
	Their Reaction	**Your Response**
IGNORE the data. (Don't even bother to "explain" data away.)	*My occupational therapy colleague glanced at the article I showed them and then changed the topic to something else.*	*Send them the article as a follow-up email and ask if we can schedule a meeting to talk about it. They might need more time to process the information.*
REJECT the data. (Articulate an explanation for why data should be rejected.)		
EXCLUDE the data from the domain of current beliefs. (The data are outside the domain of current beliefs.)		
Hold the data in ABEYANCE. (I promise to deal with it later. Assume that someday current beliefs will be articulated so that it can explain these data.)		
REINTERPRET the data while retaining current beliefs. (Accept the data as something that should be explained by current beliefs. Opposing forces accept data but interpret the data differently based on their own beliefs.)		
Reinterpret the data and MAKE PERIPHERAL CHANGES to current belief. (Make a relatively minor change to current belief; accepts the data but is unwilling to give up current belief and accept new beliefs.)		
Accept the data and CHANGE current beliefs, possibly in favor of a particular new belief. (Change one or more of the core aspects of current beliefs; when faced with information that is contradictory to current beliefs, accepts alternate beliefs.)		

References in Alphabetical Order

Balshem, H., Helfand, M., Schuneman, H. J., Oxman, A. D., Kunz, R., Brozek, J., Vist, G., Falck-Ytter, Y., Meerpohl, J., Norris, S., & Guyatt, G. H. (2011). GRADE guidelines: 3. Rating the quality of evidence. *Journal of Clinical Epidemiology, 64*, 401-406. https://doi.org/10.1016/j.jclinepi.2010.07.015

Bannigan, K., & Moores, A. (2009). A model of professional thinking: Integrating reflective practice and evidence-based practice. *Canadian Journal of Occupational Therapy, 76*(5), 342-350. https://doi.org/10.1177%2F000841740907600505

Berger, S., McAteer, J., Schreier, K., & Kaldenberg, J. (2013). Occupational therapy interventions to improve leisure and social participation for older adults with low vision: A systematic review. *American Journal of Occupational Therapy, 67*, 303-311. http://dx.doi.org/10.5014/ajot.2013.005447

Bickmore, T. W., Caruso, L., Clough-Gorr, K., & Heeren, T. (2005). "It's just like you talk to a friend" relational agents for older adults. *Interacting with Computers, 17*, 711-735. https://doi.org/10.1016/j.intcom.2005.09.002

Borenstein, M., Hedges, L., Higgins, J. & Rothstein, H. (2009). *Introduction to meta-analysis.* John Wiley & Sons, Ltd. ISBN-13: 9780470057247, online ISBN: 9780470743386, doi: 10.1002/9780470743386

Brown, C. (2016). *The evidence-based practitioner: Applying research to meet client needs* (2nd ed.). F. A. Davis Company. ISBN-10: 1719642818, ISBN-13: 9781719642811.

Bushby, K., Chan, J., Druif, S., Ho, K., & Kinsella, E. A. (2015). Ethical tensions in occupational therapy practice: A scoping review. *British Journal of Occupational Therapy, 78*(4), 212-221. https://doi.org/10.1177/0308022614564770

Campbell, R. J., & Nolfi, D. A. (2005). Teaching elderly adults to use the internet to access health care information: Before-after study. *Journal of Medical Internet Research, 7*(2), e19. https://doi.org/10.2196/jmir.7.2.e19

Chinn, C. A., & Brewer, W. F. (1993). The role of anomalous data in knowledge acquisition: A theoretical framework and implications for science instruction. *Review of Educational Research, 63*(1), 1-49. https://doi.org/10.3102/00346543063001001

Clark, G., David, K., & Woodward, G. (2006). *Progress monitoring for teachers of students who have visual disabilities.* Iowa Department of Education. https://publications.iowa.gov/6369/1/index2.pdf

Conn, A., Bourke, N., James, C., & Haracz, K. (2019). Occupational therapy intervention addressing weight gain and obesity in people with severe mental illness: A scoping review. *Australian Occupational Therapy Journal, 66*(4), 446-457. https://doi.org/10.1111/1440-1630.12575

Demeris, G., Rantz, M. J., Aud, M. A., Marek, K. D., Tyrer, H. W., Skubic, M., & Hussam, A. A. (2004). Older adults' attitudes towards and perceptions of "smart home" technologies: A pilot study. *Medical Informatics and the Internet in Medicine, 29*(2), 87-94. https://doi.org/10.1080/14639230410001684387

Dunn, W., & Proffitt, R. *Bringing Evidence Into Everyday Practice: Practical Strategies for Health Care Professionals, Second Edition* (pp. 149-152).
© 2024 Taylor & Francis Group.

DeSantis, A., Harkins, D., Tronick, E., Kaplan, E., & Beeghly, M. (2011). Exploring an integrative model of infant behavior: What is the relationship among temperament, sensory processing, and neurobehavioral measures? *Infant Behavior and Development, 34*(2), 280-292. https://doi.org/10.1016/j.infbeh.2011.01.003

Dirette, D., Rozich, A., & Viau, S. (2009). Is there enough evidence for evidence-based practice in occupational therapy? *American Journal of Occupational Therapy, 63*(6), 782-786. https://doi.org/10.5014/ajot.63.6.782

Filipova, V., Lonzaric, D., & Papez, B. J. (2015). Efficacy of combined physical and occupational therapy in patients with conservatively treated distal radius fracture: Randomized controlled trial. *Central European Journal of Medicine, 127*(Suppl. 5), S282-S287. https://doi.org/10.1007/s00508-015-0812-9

Finlayson, M., Preissner, K., Cho, C., & Plow, M. (2011). Randomization trial of a teleconference-delivered fatigue management program for people with multiple sclerosis. *Multiple Sclerosis Journal, 17*(9), 1130-1140. https://doi.org/10.1177/1352458511404272

Gellis, Z. D., Kenaley, B., McGinty, J., Bardelli, E., Davitt, J., & Ten Have, T. (2012). Outcomes of a telehealth intervention for homebound older adults with heart or chronic respiratory failure: A randomized controlled trial. *The Gerontologist, 52*(4), 541-552. https://doi.org/10.1093/geront/gnr134

Hand, C., Law, M., & McColl, M. A. (2011). Occupational therapy interventions for chronic diseases: A scoping review. *American Journal of Occupational Therapy, 65*(4), 428-436. https://doi.org/10.5014/ajot.2011.002071

He, M., Wang, Q., Zhao, J., & Wang, Y. (2021). Efficacy of ultra-early rehabilitation on elbow function after Slongo's external fixation for supracondylar humeral fractures in older children and adolescents. *Journal of Orthopedic Surgery and Research, 16*(520), e1-e7. https://doi.org/10.1186/s13018-021-02671-4

Huang, C., Yen, H., Tseng, M., Tung, L., Chen, Y., & Chen, K. (2014). Impacts of autistic behaviors, emotional and behavioral problems on parenting stress in caregivers of children with autism. *Journal of Autism and Developmental Disorders, 44*(6), 1383-1390. https://doi.org/10.1007/s10803-013-2000-y

Ikiugu, M. N., Nissen, R. M., Bellar, C., Maassen, A., & Van Peursem, K. (2017). Clinical effectiveness of occupational therapy in mental health: A meta-analysis. *American Journal of Occupational Therapy, 71*(5), 7105100020p1-7105100020p10. https://doi.org/10.5014/ajot.2017.024588

Ilott, I. (2003). Evidence-based practice forum. Challenging the rhetoric and reality: Only an individual and systemic approach will work for evidence-based occupational therapy. *American Journal of Occupational Therapy, 57*(3), 351-354. https://doi.org/10.5014/ajot.57.3.351

Kim, H., Chang, M., Rose, K., & Kim, S. (2012). Predictors of caregiver burden in caregivers of individuals with dementia. *Journal of Advanced Nursing, 68*(4), 846-855. https://doi.org/10.1111/j.1365-2648.2011.05787.x

Kitago, T., Liang, J., Huang, V. S., Hayes, S., Simon, P., Tenteromano, L., Lazar, R. M., Marshall, R. S., Mazzoni P., Lennihan, L., & Krakauer, J. W. (2013). Improvement after constraint-induced movement therapy: Recovery of normal motor control or task specific compensation? *Neurorehabilitation and Neural Repair, 27*(2), 99-109. https://doi.org/10.1177/1545968312452631

Klingels, K., Feys, H., Molenaers, G., Verbeke, G., Van Daele, S., Hoskens, J., Desloovere, K., & De Cock, P. (2013). Randomized trial of modified constraint-induced movement therapy with and without an intensive therapy program in children with unilateral cerebral palsy. *Neurorehabilitation and Neural Repair, 27*(9), 799-807. https://doi.org/10.1177/1545968313496322

Kramer, P., & Grampurohit, N. (2020). *Hinojosa and Kramer's evaluation in occupational therapy: Obtaining and interpreting data* (5th ed.). AOTA Press. ISBN-10: 1569005958; ISBN-13: 9781569005958.

Lal, S., Jarus, T., & Suto, M. J. (2012). A scoping review of the photovoice method: Implications for occupational therapy research. *Canadian Journal of Occupational Therapy, 79*(3), 181-190. https://doi.org/10.2182/cjot.2012.79.3.8

Lane, A. E., Molloy, C. A., & Bishop, S. L. (2014). Classification of children with autism spectrum disorder by sensory subtype: A case for sensory-based phenotypes. *Autism Research, 7*(3), 322-333. https://doi.org/10.1002/aur.1368

Law, M., Baptiste, S., McColl, M., Opzoomer, A., Polatajko, H., & Pollock, N. (1990). The Canadian Occupational Performance Measure: An outcome measure for occupational therapy. *Canadian Journal of Occupational Therapy, 57*(2), 82-87. doi: 10.1177/000841749005700207

Law, M., & MacDermid, J. (2014). *Evidence-based rehabilitation: A guide to practice* (3rd ed.). SLACK Incorporated. ISBN-10: 1617110213, ISBN-13: 9781617110214.

Lee, C. J., & Miller, L. T. (2003). Evidence-based practice forum. The process of evidence-based clinical decision making in occupational therapy. *American Journal of Occupational Therapy, 57*(4), 473-477. https://doi.org/10.5014/ajot.57.4.473

Little, L. M., Dean, E., Tomchek, S. D., & Dunn, W. (2016). Classifying sensory profiles of children in the general population. *Child: Care, Health and Development, 43*(1), 81-88. https://doi.org/10.1111/cch.12391

Liu, C.-J., Brost, M. A., Horton, V. E., Kenyon, S. B., & Mears, K. E. (2013). Occupational therapy interventions to improve performance of daily activities at home for older adults with low vision: A systematic review. *American Journal of Occupational Therapy, 67*, 279-287. http://dx.doi.org/10.5014/ajot.2013.005512

McWilliam, R. A. (1999). Controversial practices: The need for a re-acculturation of early intervention fields. *Topics in Early Childhood Special Education, 19*(3), 177-188. https://doi.org/10.1177%2F027112149901900310

Mendella, P. D., Burton, C. Z., Tasca, G. A., Roy, P., St. Louis, L., & Twamley, E. W. (2015). Compensatory cognitive training for people with first-episode schizophrenia: Results from a pilot randomized controlled trial. *Schizophrenia Research, 162*(1-3), 108-111. https://doi.org/10.1016/j.schres.2015.01.016

Nickel, R. E. (1996). Controversial therapies for young children with developmental disabilities. *Infants and Young Children, 8*(4), 29-40. https://doi.org/10.1097/00001163-199604000-00005

Northouse, L. L., Katapodi, M. C., Schafenacker, A. M., & Weiss, D. (2012). The impact of caregiving on the psychological well-being of family caregivers and cancer patients. *Seminars in Oncology Nursing, 28*(4), 236-245. https://doi.org/10.1016/j.soncn.2012.09.006

OCEBM Levels of Evidence Working Group*. The Oxford Levels of Evidence 2. Oxford Centre for Evidence-Based Medicine. https://www.cebm.ox.ac.uk/resources/levels-of-evidence/ocebm-levels-of-evidence

Ottenbacher, K. J., Tickle-Degnen, L., & Hasselkus, B. R. (2002). From the desk of the editor. Therapists awake! The challenge of evidence-based occupational therapy. *American Journal of Occupational Therapy, 56*(3), 247-249. https://doi.org/10.5014/ajot.56.3.247

Pankow, L., Luchins, D., Studebaker, J., & Chettleburgh, D. (2004). Evaluation of a vision rehabilitation program for older adults with visual impairment. *Topics in Geriatric Rehabilitation, 20*, 223-232.

Peiris, C. L., Shields, N., Brusco, N. K., Watts, J. J., & Taylor, N. F. (2013). Additional Saturday rehabilitation improves functional independence and quality of life and reduces length of stay: A randomized controlled trial. *BMC Medicine, 11*(1), 1-11. https://doi.org/10.1186/1741-7015-11-198

Portney, L. G. (Ed.). (2020). *Foundations of clinical research: Applications to evidence-based practice* (4th ed.). F. A. Davis Company. ISBN-10: 0803661134, ISBN-13: 9780803661134, https://fadavispt.mhmedical.com/

Portney, L. G., & Watkins, M. (2009). *Foundations of clinical research: Applications to practice* (3rd ed.). Prentice Hall. ISBN-10: 0131716409, ISBN-13: 9780131716407.

Rappolt, S. (2003). Evidence-based practice forum. The role of professional expertise in evidence-based occupational therapy. *American Journal of Occupational Therapy, 57*(5), 589-593. https://doi.org/10.5014/ajot.57.5.589

Reeder, B., Demeris, G., & Marek, K. D. (2013). Older adults' satisfaction with a medication dispensing device in home care. *Informatics for Health and Social Care, 38*(3), 211-222. https://doi.org/10.3109/17538157.2012.741084

Rix, J. (2007, October 20). *Are you a sensory junkie or a nervous wreck?* The Times. https://www.thetimes.co.uk/article/are-you-a-sensory-junkie-or-a-nervous-wreck-w8qns8rrgzw

Schwandt, M., Harris, J. E., Thomas, S., Keightley, M., Snaiderman, A., & Colantonio, A. (2012). Feasibility and effect of aerobic exercise for lowering depressive symptoms among individuals with traumatic brain injury: A pilot study. *Journal of Head Trauma Rehabilitation, 27*(2), 99-103. https://doi.org/10.1097/HTR.0b013e31820e6858

Spencer, B., Sherman, L., Nielsen, S., & Thormodson, K. (2018). Effectiveness of occupational therapy interventions for students with mental illness transitioning to higher education: A systematic review. *Occupational Therapy in Mental Health, 34*(2), 151-164. https://doi.org/10.1080/0164212X.2017.1380559

Thomas, A., & Law, M. (2013). Research utilization and evidence-based practice in occupational therapy: A scoping study. *American Journal of Occupational Therapy, 67*(4), e55-e65. https://doi.org/10.5014/ajot.2013.006395

Tickle-Degnen, L. (1999). Evidence-based practice forum. Organizing, evaluating, and using evidence. *American Journal of Occupational Therapy, 53*(6), 537-539. https://doi.org/10.5014/ajot.53.5.537

Tickle-Degnen, L. (2000a). Evidence-based practice forum. Communicating with clients, family members, and colleagues about research evidence. *American Journal of Occupational Therapy, 54*(3), 341-343. https://doi.org/10.5014/ajot.54.3.341

Tickle-Degnen, L. (2000b). Evidence-based practice forum. Gathering current research evidence to enhance clinical reasoning. *American Journal of Occupational Therapy, 54*(1), 102-105. https://doi.org/10.5014/ajot.54.1.102

Tickle-Degnen, L. (2000c). Evidence-based practice forum. Monitoring and documenting evidence during assessment and intervention. *American Journal of Occupational Therapy, 54*(4), 434-436. https://doi.org/10.5014/ajot.54.4.434

Tickle-Degnen, L. (2000d). Evidence-based practice forum. What is the best evidence to use in practice? *American Journal of Occupational Therapy, 54*(2), 218-221. https://doi.org/10.5014/ajot.54.2.218

Tickle-Degnen, L. (2001). From the general to the specific: Using meta-analytic reports in clinical decision making. *Evaluation and the Health Professions, 24*(3), 308-326. https://doi.org/10.1177/01632780122034939

Tickle-Degnen, L. (2003). Evidence-based practice forum. Where is the individual in statistics? *American Journal of Occupational Therapy, 57*(1), 112-115. https://doi.org/10.5014/ajot.57.1.112

Tickle-Degnen, L., & Bedell, G. (2003). Evidence-based practice forum. Heterarchy and hierarchy: A critical appraisal of the levels of evidence as a tool for clinical decision making. *American Journal of Occupational Therapy, 57*(2), 234-237. https://doi.org/10.5014/ajot.57.2.234

Tomchek, S., Little, L. M., Myers, J., & Dunn, W. (2018). Sensory subtypes in preschool aged children with autism spectrum disorder. *Journal of Autism and Developmental Disorders, 48*(6), 2139-2147. https://doi.org/10.1007/s10803-018-3468-2

Tomlin, G., & Borgetto, B. (2011). Research pyramid: A new evidence-based practice model for occupational therapy. *American Journal of Occupational Therapy, 65*(2), 189-196. https://doi.org/10.5014/ajot.2011.000828

Truong, V., & Hodgetts, S. (2017). An exploration of teacher perceptions toward occupational therapy and occupational therapy practices: A scoping review. *Journal of Occupational Therapy, Schools, & Early Intervention, 10*(2), 121-136. https://doi.org/10.1080/19411243.2017.1304840

Uljarevic, M., Lane, A., Kelly, A., & Leekam, S. (2016). Sensory subtypes and anxiety in older children and adolescents with autism spectrum disorder. *Autism Research, 9*(10) 1073–1078. https://doi.org/10.1002/aur.1602

Velligan, D. I., Mueller, J., Wang, M., Dicocco, M., Diamond, P. M., Maples, N. J., & Davis, B. (2006). Use of environmental supports among patients with schizophrenia. *Psychiatric Services, 57*(2), 219-224. https://doi.org/10.1176/appi.ps.57.2.219

Wallis, A., Meredith, P., & Stanley, M. (2020). Cancer care and occupational therapy: A scoping review. *Australian Occupational Therapy Journal, 67*(2), 172-194. https://doi.org/10.1111/1440-1630.12633

Wallis, C. (2007, December 10). Making sense of your senses. *Time Magazine, 170*(124).

Yusif, S., Soar, J., & Hafeez-Baig, A. (2016). Older people, assistive technologies, and the barriers to adoption: A systematic review. *International Journal of Medical Informatics, 94,* 112-116. https://doi.org/10.1016/j.ijmedinf.2016.07.004

References by Unit

Introduction

Brown, C. (2016). *The evidence-based practitioner: Applying research to meet client needs* (2nd ed.). F. A. Davis Company. ISBN-10: 1719642818, ISBN-13: 9781719642811.

Law, M., & MacDermid, J. (2014). *Evidence-based rehabilitation: A guide to practice* (3rd ed.). SLACK Incorporated. ISBN-10: 1617110213, ISBN-13: 9781617110214.

Portney, L. G. (Ed.). (2020). *Foundations of clinical research: Applications to evidence-based practice* (4th ed.). F. A. Davis Company. ISBN-10: 0803661134, ISBN-13: 9780803661134, https://fadavispt.mhmedical.com/

Unit 1

Balshem, H., Helfand, M., Schuneman, H. J., Oxman, A. D., Kunz, R., Brozek, J., Vist, G., Falck-Ytter, Y., Meerpohl, J., Norris, S., & Guyatt, G. H. (2011). GRADE guidelines: 3. Rating the quality of evidence. *Journal of Clinical Epidemiology, 64*, 401-406. https://doi.org/10.1016/j.jclinepi.2010.07.015

Bannigan, K., & Moores, A. (2009). A model of professional thinking: Integrating reflective practice and evidence-based practice. *Canadian Journal of Occupational Therapy, 76*(5), 342-350. https://doi.org/10.1177%2F000841740907600505

Brown, C. (2016). *The evidence-based practitioner: Applying research to meet client needs* (2nd ed.). F. A. Davis Company. ISBN-10: 1719642818, ISBN-13: 9781719642811.

Dirette, D., Rozich, A., & Viau, S. (2009). Is there enough evidence for evidence-based practice in occupational therapy? *American Journal of Occupational Therapy, 63*(6), 782-786. https://doi.org/10.5014/ajot.63.6.782

Ilott, I. (2003). Evidence-based practice forum. Challenging the rhetoric and reality: Only an individual and systemic approach will work for evidence-based occupational therapy. *American Journal of Occupational Therapy, 57*(3), 351-354. https://doi.org/10.5014/ajot.57.3.351

Law, M., & MacDermid, J. (2014). *Evidence-based rehabilitation: A guide to practice* (3rd ed.). SLACK Incorporated. ISBN-10: 1617110213, ISBN-13: 9781617110214.

Dunn, W., & Proffitt, R. *Bringing Evidence Into Everyday Practice: Practical Strategies for Health Care Professionals, Second Edition* (pp. 153-158). © 2024 Taylor & Francis Group.

Lee, C. J., & Miller, L. T. (2003). Evidence-based practice forum. The process of evidence-based clinical decision making in occupational therapy. *American Journal of Occupational Therapy, 57*(4), 473-477. https://doi.org/10.5014/ajot.57.4.473

OCEBM Levels of Evidence Working Group*. The Oxford Levels of Evidence 2. Oxford Centre for Evidence-Based Medicine. https://www.cebm.ox.ac.uk/resources/levels-of-evidence/ocebm-levels-of-evidence

Ottenbacher, K. J., Tickle-Degnen, L., & Hasselkus, B. R. (2002). From the desk of the editor. Therapists awake! The challenge of evidence-based occupational therapy. *American Journal of Occupational Therapy, 56*(3), 247-249. https://doi.org/10.5014/ajot.56.3.247

Portney, L. G. (Ed.). (2020). *Foundations of clinical research: Applications to evidence-based practice* (4th ed.). F. A. Davis Company. ISBN-10: 0803661134, ISBN-13: 9780803661134, https://fadavispt.mhmedical.com/

Rappolt, S. (2003). Evidence-based practice forum. The role of professional expertise in evidence-based occupational therapy. *American Journal of Occupational Therapy, 57*(5), 589-593. https://doi.org/10.5014/ajot.57.5.589

Tickle-Degnen, L. (1999). Evidence-based practice forum. Organizing, evaluating, and using evidence. *American Journal of Occupational Therapy, 53*(6), 537-539. https://doi.org/10.5014/ajot.53.5.537

Tickle-Degnen, L. (2000a). Evidence-based practice forum. Communicating with clients, family members, and colleagues about research evidence. *American Journal of Occupational Therapy, 54*(3), 341-343. https://doi.org/10.5014/ajot.54.3.341

Tickle-Degnen, L. (2000b). Evidence-based practice forum. Gathering current research evidence to enhance clinical reasoning. *American Journal of Occupational Therapy, 54*(1), 102-105. https://doi.org/10.5014/ajot.54.1.102

Tickle-Degnen, L. (2000c). Evidence-based practice forum. Monitoring and documenting evidence during assessment and intervention. *American Journal of Occupational Therapy, 54*(4), 434-436. https://doi.org/10.5014/ajot.54.4.434

Tickle-Degnen, L. (2000d). Evidence-based practice forum. What is the best evidence to use in practice? *American Journal of Occupational Therapy, 54*(2), 218-221. https://doi.org/10.5014/ajot.54.2.218

Tickle-Degnen, L. (2003). Evidence-based practice forum. Where is the individual in statistics? *American Journal of Occupational Therapy, 57*(1), 112-115. https://doi.org/10.5014/ajot.57.1.112

Tickle-Degnen, L., & Bedell, G. (2003). Evidence-based practice forum. Heterarchy and hierarchy: A critical appraisal of the levels of evidence as a tool for clinical decision making. *American Journal of Occupational Therapy, 57*(2), 234-237. https://doi.org/10.5014/ajot.57.2.234

Thomas, A., & Law, M. (2013). Research utilization and evidence-based practice in occupational therapy: A scoping study. *American Journal of Occupational Therapy, 67*(4), e55-e65. https://doi.org/10.5014/ajot.2013.006395

Tomlin, G., & Borgetto, B. (2011). Research pyramid: A new evidence-based practice model for occupational therapy. *American Journal of Occupational Therapy, 65*(2), 189-196. https://doi.org/10.5014/ajot.2011.000828

UNIT 2

Chinn, C. A., & Brewer, W. F. (1993). The role of anomalous data in knowledge acquisition: A theoretical framework and implications for science instruction. *Review of Educational Research, 63*(1), 1-49. https://doi.org/10.3102/00346543063001001

Unit 3

Berger, S., McAteer, J., Schreier, K., & Kaldenberg, J. (2013). Occupational therapy interventions to improve leisure and social participation for older adults with low vision: A systematic review. *American Journal of Occupational Therapy, 67,* 303-311. http://dx.doi.org/10.5014/ajot.2013.005447

Chinn, C. A., & Brewer, W. F. (1993). The role of anomalous data in knowledge acquisition: A theoretical framework and implications for science instruction. *Review of Educational Research, 63*(1), 1-49. https://doi.org/10.3102/00346543063001001

Finlayson, M., Preissner, K., Cho, C., & Plow, M. (2011). Randomization trial of a teleconference-delivered fatigue management program for people with multiple sclerosis. *Multiple Sclerosis Journal, 17*(9), 1130-1140. https://doi.org/10.1177/1352458511404272

Kramer, P., & Grampurohit, N. (2020). *Hinojosa and Kramer's evaluation in occupational therapy: Obtaining and interpreting data* (5th ed.). AOTA Press. ISBN-10: 1569005958; ISBN-13: 9781569005958.

Law, M., & MacDermid, J. (2014). *Evidence-based rehabilitation: A guide to practice* (3rd ed.). SLACK Incorporated. ISBN-10: 1617110213, ISBN-13: 9781617110214.

Liu, C.-J., Brost, M. A., Horton, V. E., Kenyon, S. B., & Mears, K. E. (2013). Occupational therapy interventions to improve performance of daily activities at home for older adults with low vision: A systematic review. *American Journal of Occupational Therapy, 67,* 279-287. http://dx.doi.org/10.5014/ajot.2013.005512

Pankow, L., Luchins, D., Studebaker, J., & Chettleburgh, D. (2004). Evaluation of a vision rehabilitation program for older adults with visual impairment. *Topics in Geriatric Rehabilitation, 20,* 223-232.

Peiris, C. L., Shields, N., Brusco, N. K., Watts, J. J., & Taylor, N. F. (2013). Additional Saturday rehabilitation improves functional independence and quality of life and reduces length of stay: A randomized controlled trial. *BMC Medicine, 11*(1), 1-11. https://doi.org/10.1186/1741-7015-11-198

Portney, L. G. (Ed.). (2020). *Foundations of clinical research: Applications to evidence-based practice* (4th ed.). F. A. Davis Company. ISBN-10: 0803661134, ISBN-13: 9780803661134, https://fadavispt.mhmedical.com/

Schwandt, M., Harris, J. E., Thomas, S., Keightley, M., Snaiderman, A., & Colantonio, A. (2012). Feasibility and effect of aerobic exercise for lowering depressive symptoms among individuals with traumatic brain injury: A pilot study. *Journal of Head Trauma Rehabilitation, 27*(2), 99-103. https://doi.org/10.1097/HTR.0b013e31820e6858

Unit 4

Bickmore, T. W., Caruso, L., Clough-Gorr, K., & Heeren, T. (2005). "It's just like you talk to a friend" relational agents for older adults. *Interacting with Computers, 17,* 711-735. https://doi.org/10.1016/j.intcom.2005.09.002

Campbell, R. J., & Nolfi, D. A. (2005). Teaching elderly adults to use the internet to access health care information: Before-after study. *Journal of Medical Internet Research, 7*(2), e19. https://doi.org/10.2196/jmir.7.2.e19

Chinn, C. A., & Brewer, W. F. (1993). The role of anomalous data in knowledge acquisition: A theoretical framework and implications for science instruction. *Review of Educational Research, 63*(1), 1-49. https://doi.org/10.3102/00346543063001001

Demeris, G., Rantz, M. J., Aud, M. A., Marek, K. D., Tyrer, H. W., Skubic, M., & Hussam, A. A. (2004). Older adults' attitudes towards and perceptions of "smart home" technologies: A pilot study. *Medical Informatics and the Internet in Medicine, 29*(2), 87-94. https://doi.org/10.1080/14639230410001684387

Gellis, Z. D., Kenaley, B., McGinty, J., Bardelli, E., Davitt, J., & Ten Have, T. (2012). Outcomes of a telehealth intervention for homebound older adults with heart or chronic respiratory failure: A randomized controlled trial. *The Gerontologist, 52*(4), 541-552. https://doi.org/10.1093/geront/gnr134

Reeder, B., Demeris, G., & Marek, K. D. (2013). Older adults' satisfaction with a medication dispensing device in home care. *Informatics for Health and Social Care, 38*(3), 211-222. https://doi.org/10.3109/17538157.2012.741084

Yusif, S., Soar, J., & Hafeez-Baig, A. (2016). Older people, assistive technologies, and the barriers to adoption: A systematic review. *International Journal of Medical Informatics, 94,* 112-116. https://doi.org/10.1016/j.ijmedinf.2016.07.004

Unit 5

Chinn, C. A., & Brewer, W. F. (1993). The role of anomalous data in knowledge acquisition: A theoretical framework and implications for science instruction. *Review of Educational Research, 63*(1), 1-49. https://doi.org/10.3102/00346543063001001

Mendella, P. D., Burton, C. Z., Tasca, G. A., Roy, P., St. Louis, L., & Twamley, E. W. (2015). Compensatory cognitive training for people with first-episode schizophrenia: Results from a pilot randomized controlled trial. *Schizophrenia Research, 162*(1-3), 108-111. https://doi.org/10.1016/j.schres.2015.01.016

Velligan, D. I., Mueller, J., Wang, M., Dicocco, M., Diamond, P. M., Maples, N. J., & Davis, B. (2006). Use of environmental supports among patients with schizophrenia. *Psychiatric Services, 57*(2), 219-224. https://doi.org/10.1176/appi.ps.57.2.219

Unit 6

Chinn, C. A., & Brewer, W. F. (1993). The role of anomalous data in knowledge acquisition: A theoretical framework and implications for science instruction. *Review of Educational Research, 63*(1), 1-49. https://doi.org/10.3102/00346543063001001

Huang, C., Yen, H., Tseng, M., Tung, L., Chen, Y., & Chen, K. (2014). Impacts of autistic behaviors, emotional and behavioral problems on parenting stress in caregivers of children with autism. *Journal of Autism and Developmental Disorders, 44*(6), 1383-1390. https://doi.org/10.1007/s10803-013-2000-y

Kim, H., Chang, M., Rose, K., & Kim, S. (2012). Predictors of caregiver burden in caregivers of individuals with dementia. *Journal of Advanced Nursing, 68*(4), 846-855. https://doi.org/10.1111/j.1365-2648.2011.05787.x

Northouse, L. L., Katapodi, M. C., Schafenacker, A. M., & Weiss, D. (2012). The impact of caregiving on the psychological well-being of family caregivers and cancer patients. *Seminars in Oncology Nursing, 28*(4), 236-245. https://doi.org/10.1016/j.soncn.2012.09.006

Unit 7

Chinn, C. A., & Brewer, W. F. (1993). The role of anomalous data in knowledge acquisition: A theoretical framework and implications for science instruction. *Review of Educational Research, 63*(1), 1-49. https://doi.org/10.3102/00346543063001001

DeSantis, A., Harkins, D., Tronick, E., Kaplan, E., & Beeghly, M. (2011). Exploring an integrative model of infant behavior: What is the relationship among temperament, sensory processing, and neurobehavioral measures? *Infant Behavior and Development, 34*(2), 280-292. https://doi.org/10.1016/j.infbeh.2011.01.003

Lane, A. E., Molloy, C. A., & Bishop, S. L. (2014). Classification of children with autism spectrum disorder by sensory subtype: A case for sensory-based phenotypes. *Autism Research, 7*(3), 322-333. https://doi.org/10.1002/aur.1368

Little, L. M., Dean, E., Tomchek, S. D., & Dunn, W. (2016). Classifying sensory profiles of children in the general population. *Child: Care, Health and Development, 43*(1), 81-88. https://doi.org/10.1111/cch.12391

Rix, J. (2007, October 20). *Are you a sensory junkie or a nervous wreck?* The Times. https://www.thetimes.co.uk/article/are-you-a-sensory-junkie-or-a-nervous-wreck-w8qns8rrgzw

Tomchek, S., Little, L. M., Myers, J., & Dunn, W. (2018). Sensory subtypes in preschool aged children with autism spectrum disorder. *Journal of Autism and Developmental Disorders, 48*(6), 2139-2147. https://doi.org/10.1007/s10803-018-3468-2

Uljarevic, M., Lane, A., Kelly, A., & Leekam, S. (2016). Sensory subtypes and anxiety in older children and adolescents with autism spectrum disorder. *Autism Research, 9*(10) 1073–1078. https://doi.org/10.1002/aur.1602

Wallis, C. (2007, December 10). Making sense of your senses. *Time Magazine, 170*(124).

UNIT 8

Chinn, C. A., & Brewer, W. F. (1993). The role of anomalous data in knowledge acquisition: A theoretical framework and implications for science instruction. *Review of Educational Research, 63*(1), 1-49. https://doi. org/10.3102/00346543063001001

Kitago, T., Liang, J., Huang, V. S., Hayes, S., Simon, P., Tenteromano, L., Lazar, R. M., Marshall, R. S., Mazzoni P., Lennihan, L., & Krakauer, J. W. (2013). Improvement after constraint-induced movement therapy: Recovery of normal motor control or task specific compensation? *Neurorehabilitation and Neural Repair, 27*(2), 99-109. https://doi.org/10.1177/1545968312452631

Klingels, K., Feys, H., Molenaers, G., Verbeke, G., Van Daele, S., Hoskens, J., Desloovere, K., & De Cock, P. (2013). Randomized trial of modified constraint-induced movement therapy with and without an intensive therapy program in children with unilateral cerebral palsy. *Neurorehabilitation and Neural Repair, 27*(9), 799-807. https://doi.org/10.1177/1545968313496322

UNIT 9

Chinn, C. A., & Brewer, W. F. (1993). The role of anomalous data in knowledge acquisition: A theoretical framework and implications for science instruction. *Review of Educational Research, 63*(1), 1-49. https://doi. org/10.3102/00346543063001001

Filipova, V., Lonzaric, D., & Papez, B. J. (2015). Efficacy of combined physical and occupational therapy in patients with conservatively treated distal radius fracture: Randomized controlled trial. *Central European Journal of Medicine, 127*(Suppl. 5), S282-S287. https://doi.org/10.1007/s00508-015-0812-9

He, M., Wang, Q., Zhao, J., & Wang, Y. (2021). Efficacy of ultra-early rehabilitation on elbow function after Slongo's external fixation for supracondylar humeral fractures in older children and adolescents. *Journal of Orthopedic Surgery and Research, 16*(520), e1-e7. https://doi.org/10.1186/s13018-021-02671-4

Portney, L. G. (Ed.). (2020). *Foundations of clinical research: Applications to evidence-based practice* (4th ed.). F. A. Davis Company. ISBN-10: 0803661134, ISBN-13: 9780803661134, https://fadavispt.mhmedical.com/

Portney, L. G., & Watkins, M. (2009). *Foundations of clinical research: Applications to practice* (3rd ed.). Prentice Hall. ISBN-10: 0131716409, ISBN-13: 9780131716407.

Tickle-Degnen, L. (2001). From the general to the specific: Using meta-analytic reports in clinical decision making. *Evaluation and the Health Professions, 24*(3), 308-326. https://doi.org/10.1177/01632780122034939

UNIT 10

Borenstein, M., Hedges, L., Higgins, J. & Rothstein, H. (2009). *Introduction to meta-analysis.* John Wiley & Sons, Ltd. ISBN-13: 9780470057247, online ISBN: 9780470743386, doi: 10.1002/9780470743386

Bushby, K., Chan, J., Druif, S., Ho, K., & Kinsella, E. A. (2015). Ethical tensions in occupational therapy practice: A scoping review. *British Journal of Occupational Therapy, 78*(4), 212-221. https://doi. org/10.1177/0308022614564770

Conn, A., Bourke, N., James, C., & Haracz, K. (2019). Occupational therapy intervention addressing weight gain and obesity in people with severe mental illness: A scoping review. *Australian Occupational Therapy Journal, 66*(4), 446-457. https://doi.org/10.1111/1440-1630.12575

Hand, C., Law, M., & McColl, M. A. (2011). Occupational therapy interventions for chronic diseases: A scoping review. *American Journal of Occupational Therapy, 65*(4), 428-436. https://doi.org/10.5014/ajot.2011.002071

Ikiugu, M. N., Nissen, R. M., Bellar, C., Maassen, A., & Van Peursem, K. (2017). Clinical effectiveness of occupational therapy in mental health: A meta-analysis. *American Journal of Occupational Therapy, 71*(5), 7105100020p1-7105100020p10. https://doi.org/10.5014/ajot.2017.024588

Lal, S., Jarus, T., & Suto, M. J. (2012). A scoping review of the photovoice method: Implications for occupational therapy research. *Canadian Journal of Occupational Therapy, 79*(3), 181-190. https://doi.org/10.2182/cjot.2012.79.3.8

Portney, L. G. (Ed.). (2020). *Foundations of clinical research: Applications to evidence-based practice* (4th ed.). F. A. Davis Company. ISBN-10: 0803661134, ISBN-13: 9780803661134, https://fadavispt.mhmedical.com/

Portney, L. G., & Watkins, M. (2009). *Foundations of clinical research: Applications to practice* (3rd ed.). Prentice Hall. ISBN-10: 0131716409, ISBN-13: 9780131716407.

Spencer, B., Sherman, L., Nielsen, S., & Thormodson, K. (2018). Effectiveness of occupational therapy interventions for students with mental illness transitioning to higher education: A systematic review. *Occupational Therapy in Mental Health, 34*(2), 151-164. https://doi.org/10.1080/0164212X.2017.1380559

Tickle-Degnen, L. (2001). From the general to the specific: Using meta-analytic reports in clinical decision making. *Evaluation and the Health Professions, 24*(3), 308-326. https://doi.org/10.1177/01632780122034939

Truong, V., & Hodgetts, S. (2017). An exploration of teacher perceptions toward occupational therapy and occupational therapy practices: A scoping review. *Journal of Occupational Therapy, Schools, & Early Intervention, 10*(2), 121-136. https://doi.org/10.1080/19411243.2017.1304840

Wallis, A., Meredith, P., & Stanley, M. (2020). Cancer care and occupational therapy: A scoping review. *Australian Occupational Therapy Journal, 67*(2), 172-194. https://doi.org/10.1111/1440-1630.12633

UNIT 11

Chinn, C. A., & Brewer, W. F. (1993). The role of anomalous data in knowledge acquisition: A theoretical framework and implications for science instruction. *Review of Educational Research, 63*(1), 1-49. https://doi.org/10.3102/00346543063001001

McWilliam, R. A. (1999). Controversial practices: The need for a re-acculturation of early intervention fields. *Topics in Early Childhood Special Education, 19*(3), 177-188. https://doi.org/10.1177%2F027112149901900310

Nickel, R. E. (1996). Controversial therapies for young children with developmental disabilities. *Infants and Young Children, 8*(4), 29-40. https://doi.org/10.1097/00001163-199604000-00005

UNIT 12

Clark, G., David, K., & Woodward, G. (2006). *Progress monitoring for teachers of students who have visual disabilities.* Iowa Department of Education. https://publications.iowa.gov/6369/1/index2.pdf

Law, M., Baptiste, S., McColl, M., Opzoomer, A., Polatajko, H., & Pollock, N. (1990). The Canadian Occupational Performance Measure: An outcome measure for occupational therapy. *Canadian Journal of Occupational Therapy, 57*(2), 82-87. doi: 10.1177/000841749005700207

UNIT 13

Chinn, C. A., & Brewer, W. F. (1993). The role of anomalous data in knowledge acquisition: A theoretical framework and implications for science instruction. *Review of Educational Research, 63*(1), 1-49. https://doi.org/10.3102/00346543063001001

Law, M., & MacDermid, J. (2014). *Evidence-based rehabilitation: A guide to practice* (3rd ed.). SLACK Incorporated. ISBN-10: 1617110213, ISBN-13: 9781617110214.

INDEX

assistive devices

anomalous data, handling, 32

assistive devices, expanding knowledge about, worksheet, 33–34

characteristics of discussion, summarizing, worksheet, 32

discussion of methods/results, extending knowledge about, 33

evidence, expanding, 32

experimental/descriptive data, combining, 33–35

findings, discussion of, 32

ideas, discussion of, 31

literature, reading, 30

organizing themes, discussion of, 34

patterns/themes, looking for, 31–32

questions, answerable/unanswerable, worksheet, 31

reactions to, new data, worksheet, 32

smart devices, 35

worksheet, 35

strengths/limitations, recognizing, 31

take-home messages, 34

creation, worksheet, 34

background knowledge, 1–26

basic parts of research articles, 13–26

entire article

introduction, 21–22

practice with, 20–26

findings from discussion of study, summarizing, 18–20

literature, reading, 14

methods/results, reviewing, 16–17

caregiving

anomalous data, handling, 45

characteristics of discussion, summarizing, worksheet, 44

conceptual themes, similarities in, worksheet, 47

evidence, expanding, 45

evidence related to, 43–48

methods/results, extending knowledge about, 46

patterns/themes, looking for, 44–46

varied studies, evidence from, 46–48

ideas, discussion of, 46

literature, reading, 44

methods/results, summarizing, 44

questions, answerable/unanswerable, worksheet, 45

strengths/limitations, recognizing, 45

take-home messages, 47–48

themes, 47

identification of, 47

unique themes across studies, finding, worksheet, 47

communicating evidence, 107–112

comparing/contrasting, 108

new data

reactions to, worksheet, 110

response to, worksheet, 111

patterns/themes, looking for, 108–112

practice, 109–112

reactions from others, 111

reactions to new data, response to, 148

responding to reactions from others, 111

take-home message, reviewing, 108, 110

take-home messages, 109–110

comparing/ contrasting, worksheet, 108

creation, worksheet, 109–110

compensatory strategies, 37–42

literature, reading, 37–38

methods/results, summarizing, 38

patterns/themes, 38–40

constraint-induced therapy interventions, 57–64

compare intervention programs, worksheet, 62

familiar measures, understanding, 61

features of interventions, comparing, 62

interventions, learning more about, 62–63

literature, reading, 58
methods/results
    extending knowledge about, 60
    summarizing, 58
patterns/themes, looking for, 58–60
practice, 61
public knowledge, 62
tables/figures, data discussion in, 60–61
take-home messages, 63
    creation, worksheet, 63
controversial practices, 91–93
anomalous data, handling, 91
evidence related to, 89–94
    key points, summarizing, 90–94
group discussion, 94
literature, reading, 90
new data, reactions to, worksheet, 91
patterns/themes, 93–94
summarizing, 90
summarizing key points for analysis,
    worksheet, 93–94
take-home messages, 94
    creation, worksheet, 94
worksheet, 91–93

databases, searching, 7

emerging practices, 91–93
anomalous data, handling, 91
evidence related to, 89–94
    key points, summarizing, 90–94
group discussion, 94
literature, reading, 90
new data, reactions to, worksheet, 91
patterns/themes, 93–94
summarizing, 90
summarizing key points for analysis,
    worksheet, 93–94
take-home messages, 94
    creation, worksheet, 94
entire article, practice with
anomalous data, 25
characteristics, summarizing discussion of
    research, worksheet, 21
decoding text results, 23–24

discussion, 24–25
    linking with results, 25
framework for study, 21
graphs/tables/text, understanding
    relationship among, 23
inclusion criteria, summarizing, 22
    worksheet, 22
introduction, examining, 21
introduction themes, summarizing,
    worksheet, 21
literature, summarizing, 21
measures, 22
    finding more information about,
        22–23
methods section of article, analyzing, 22
participants, 22
procedures, 22
research questions, 24–25
tables/figures, finding text to match, 23–24
take-home messages, 25–26
    creating, worksheet, 25–26
text of results, discussion of, 24
themes, identification of, 21
environmental adaptations
anomalous data, handling, 32
assistive devices, expanding knowledge
    about, worksheet, 33–34
assistive devices/environmental adaptations
    discussion of methods/results,
        extending knowledge about, 33
    patterns/themes, looking for, 31–32
characteristics of discussion, summarizing,
    worksheet, 32
evidence, expanding, 32
experimental/descriptive data, combining,
    33–35
findings, discussion of, 32
ideas, discussion of, 31
literature, reading, 30
organizing themes, discussion of, 34
questions, answerable/unanswerable,
    worksheet, 31
reactions to, new data, worksheet, 32
smart devices, 35
    worksheet, 35
strengths/limitations, recognizing, 31
take-home messages, 34
    creation, worksheet, 34
expanding knowledge/skills, 75–112

factors/samples, summarizing, 51
figures, text to match, finding, 23–24
figures/tables, text to match, finding, 23–24
findings from discussion of study
    linking, 40–41
    questions, worksheet, 20
    sharing with study partners, 19
    strengths/limitations, recognizing, 20
    take-home messages, 18–19
        writing, worksheet, 18–19

ideas, discussion of, 39–40
interdisciplinary issue, evidence-based practice
    as, 6–7
    comparing/contrasting, 6–7
    discussion, 7
    professional databases
        searching, 7
        searching in, 7

language of evidence-based practice, 4–6
    application of findings to practice, 5
    listing evidence-based practice concepts,
        worksheet, 5
    listing steps in implementing evidence-
        based practice, worksheet, 5
    literature, 5
    selection/reflection, 5–6
linking discussion with results, 25
literature, discussion of, 52, 60. *See also*
    discussion

meta-analysis, 77–88
    abstract, dissecting, 79
    analysis of discussion, 85–86
    critiquing authors' ideas, 81–82
    discussion of, 78–82
    examine methods, 79
    flow charts, making, 80
    graphs/findings, review of, 81
    limitations of study, 82
    literature selection, flow chart, 80
    objective, 78
    purpose of article, examining, 86–87
    relevance of study, 83

review articles, 83–84
search terms, finding, 79–80
study results, 80
take-home messages
    identification of, 82
    worksheet, 82

new concepts, identification of, 4
    discussion, 4
    familiar research concepts, identification
        of, worksheet, 4
    literature, reading, 4
    new research concepts, identification,
        worksheet, 4

own practice, creating evidence within
    discussion of, 95–106
    chart/graph, design, discussion of, 103
    data discussion, structure for, 96
    discussion of collection methods, 98–100
    graphing progress, 101–102
    measures, 96–97
    practice, 98–99, 101–104
    progress monitoring plan, worksheet, 102
    recording outcomes in context, 104–105
    recording performance and satisfaction
        with performance, 105
    scale for outcome attainment, specific,
        discussion of, 103–104

participant criteria discussion
    examining, 15
    inclusion/exclusion criteria, learning about,
        15
patterns/themes
    anomalous data, handling, 39, 52, 59
    characteristics of discussion, summarizing,
        worksheet, 59
    material, discussion of, 52, 60
    new data, reactions to, worksheet, 39, 52,
        59
    questions
        identifying, worksheet, 51, 59
        worksheet, 39
    strengths/limitations, recognizing, 39, 51,
        59

populations, linking evidence across, 40
  take-home messages, 40–41
    creation, worksheet, 40–41
  themes across studies, worksheet, 40
practice, 27–74
processing patterns, 49–56
  methods/results, extending knowledge
    about, 52–55
  patterns/themes, 51–52
public knowledge, 54
purpose of article
  new data, reactions to, worksheet, 87
  practice, application of, findings to, 86–87
  responses to findings, 87
  specific situation, application of evidence to
    discussion, worksheet, 86–87
  structure of review, reviewing, 86
  take-home messages, 87
    creation, worksheet, 87
  websites, legitimate, use of, 87

quality of evidence, determining, 8
  comparing/contrasting, 8
  evidence classification systems, comparing,
    worksheet, 8

relevance of study
  practice, application of, 83
  specific situation, application of evidence to
    discussion, worksheet, 83
responses to evidence, characterizing, 9–12
  anomalous data, ways to handle, 10–12
results
  factors/profiles, comparing features of, 53
  intervention studies, summarizing,
    worksheet, 16–17
  key points, summarizing, 16
  methods/results, summarizing, 16–17
  practice, 53
  rationale for summary points from article,
    worksheet, 53
  summary tables, similarities/differences in,
    worksheet, 16
  take-home messages, 54
review articles
  flow charts, reviewing, 84
  search parameters
    in discussion of summary study, 84
    identification of, 84

samples, summarizing, 51
sensory processing patterns, summary table for,
  worksheet, 53
skills, expanding, 75–112
smart devices, 35
  worksheet, 35
summary article, 77–88
  analysis of discussion, 85–86
    literature formats, comparing/
      contrasting, 86
  meta-analysis, 78–82
  purpose of article, examining, 86–87
  relevance of study, 83
  review articles, 83–84

tables, text to match, finding, 23–24
tables/figures, text to match, finding, 23–24
thematic analysis
  practice, application of, findings to, 85
  specific situation, application of evidence to
    discussion, worksheet, 85
tracing factors/profiles, from infancy to
  adolescence, 54

upper extremity fractures
  anomalous data, handling, 67
  evidence, expanding, 67
  evidence related to, 65–74
    patterns/themes, looking for, 66–68
  graphs from tables, 68–70
  group discussion, 68
  literature, reading, 65–66
  methods/results
    extending knowledge about, 68–71
    summarizing, 66
  new data, reactions to, worksheet, 67
  practice, 70–72
  questions, identifying, worksheet, 67
  strengths/limitations, recognizing, 67
  take-home messages, 73
    worksheet, 73
  technical wording in results,
    understanding, 72–73

websites, legitimate, use of, 87

Printed in the United States
by Baker & Taylor Publisher Services